PSYCHOTHERAPY
in CLINICAL PRACTICE

Integrating Psychological and Biological Therapies

PSYCHOTHERAPY
in CLINICAL PRACTICE

Integrating Psychological and Biological Therapies

PSYCHOTHERAPY
in CLINICAL PRACTICE

Integrating Psychological and Biological Therapies

SHEILA M. DOWD, PhD
Assistant Professor
Department of Psychiatry and Behavioral Sciences
Associate Director of Residency Training
Co-Director of the Adult Outpatient Clinic
Department of Psychiatry
Rush University Medical Center
Chicago, Illinois

PHILIP G. JANICAK, MD
Professor of Psychiatry
Rush University Medical Center
Chicago, Illinois

Wolters Kluwer | Lippincott Williams & Wilkins
Health
Philadelphia · Baltimore · New York · London
Buenos Aires · Hong Kong · Sydney · Tokyo

Acquisitions Editor: Charley Mitchell
Managing Editor: Sirkka Howes
Project Manager: Cindy Oberle
Manufacturing Manager: Kathleen Brown
Marketing Manager: Sharon Zinner
Design Coordinator: Holly Reid-McLaughlin
Production Services: Laserwords Private Limited, Chennai, India

WM
400
D745i
2009

© 2009 by LIPPINCOTT WILLIAMS & WILKINS, a WOLTERS KLUWER business
530 Walnut Street
Philadelphia, PA 19106 USA
LWW.com

Printed in the USA

Library of Congress Cataloging-in-Publication Data
Dowd, Sheila M.
  Integrating psychological and biological therapies / Sheila M. Dowd, Philip G. Janicak.
    p. ; cm.
  Includes bibliographical references and index.
  ISBN-13: 978-0-7817-5102-5
  ISBN-10: 0-7817-5102-0
  1. Biological psychiatry. 2. Psychotherapy. I. Janicak, Philip G. II. Title.
  [DNLM: 1. Mental Disorders—therapy—Case Reports. 2. Drug Therapy—methods—Case Reports. 3. Electroconvulsive Therapy—methods—Case Reports.
4. Psychotherapy—methods—Case Reports. WM 400 D745i 2008]
  RC343.D69 2008
  616.89'14—dc22

                                                            2008021293

Care has been taken to confirm the accuracy of the information presented and to describe generally accepted practices. However, the authors, editors, and publisher are not responsible for errors or omissions or for any consequences from application of the information in this book and make no warranty, expressed or implied, with respect to the currency, completeness, or accuracy of the contents of the publication. Application of the information in a particular situation remains the professional responsibility of the practitioner.

The authors, editors, and publisher have exerted every effort to ensure that drug selection and dosage set forth in this text are in accordance with current recommendations and practice at the time of publication. However, in view of ongoing research, changes in government regulations, and the constant flow of information relating to drug therapy and drug reactions, the reader is urged to check the package insert for each drug for any change in indications and dosage and for added warnings and precautions. This is particularly important when the recommended agent is a new or infrequently employed drug.

Some drugs and medical devices presented in the publication have Food and Drug Administration (FDA) clearance for limited use in restricted research settings. It is the responsibility of health care provider to ascertain the FDA status of each drug or device planned for use in their clinical practice.

To purchase additional copies of this book, call our customer service department at (800) 638-3030 or fax orders to (301) 223-2320. International customers should call (301) 223-2300.

Visit Lippincott Williams & Wilkins on the Internet: at LWW.com. Lippincott Williams & Wilkins customer service representatives are available from 8:30 AM to 6 PM, EST.

10 9 8 7 6 5 4 3 2 1

Acknowledgments

We would like to acknowledge our administrative assistant, Sandra M. Smith, who edited and organized multiple drafts of this book. Special thanks to Charley Mitchell for recognizing the importance of this topic and also to Jennifer LaGreca and Sirkka Howes whose publishing expertise brought this to fruition.

Acknowledgments

Contents

Overview

The combination of psychotherapy plus biological therapies (i.e., pharmacotherapy, device-based therapies) is frequently used to treat psychiatric disorders. In support, various studies (e.g., neurophysiological, neuroendocrine, neuroimaging) report similar actions with each approach and possibly additive or synergistic actions with combined medication and psychotherapy.[1] Further, Hollen and Fawcett[2] note that combining these treatments increases the magnitude and probability of a response, enhances the breadth of response, and improves patients' acceptance. Therefore, their careful integration is often required to achieve an optimal outcome. In this context, several combination or sequencing strategies can be considered, including:

- *Adding medication* to psychotherapy to enable the therapeutic process to proceed optimally (e.g., enhance concentration, reduce distorted thinking, reduce anxiety)
- *Adding psychotherapy* to medication to enable the therapeutic process to proceed optimally (e.g., improve patients' understanding, acceptance, and management of their illness)
- *Combining both from the outset* in disorders clearly benefited by such an approach (e.g., use psychotherapy to manage psychosocial stressors not addressed by pharmacotherapy alone)
- *Transitioning* from one approach to another in the face of issues such as *poor tolerability* or *patient preference*
- *Transitioning* from combined treatment to a single approach for *maintenance therapy* after acute symptoms are controlled

■ Utilizing psychotherapy to enhance *medication adherence* and *to prevent relapse*

It should also be noted that there is the potential risk for negative consequences when combining treatments (e.g., benzodiazepines causing dependency or interfering with learning and memory, psychotherapy producing higher stress in patients with schizophrenia).

Although major depressive disorder (MDD), obsessive compulsive disorder (OCD), various anxiety-related (e.g., panic disorder and posttraumatic stress disorder) and sleep-related problems are the best studied conditions in the context of combining therapies, there is a growing literature to support an integrated approach in such diverse conditions as schizophrenia, bipolar disorder, and borderline personality. While there are also data and clinical experience with combined treatments for conditions such as social phobia, the specific disorders covered in this book were chosen because they clearly illustrate the benefits of integrated therapy.

Considering all these issues, we will develop a series of treatment strategies to highlight the discussion of combined treatment approaches for specific diagnoses. The three underlying assumptions guiding these strategies are the best *available evidence* (primarily from adequately controlled trials), the breadth of *clinical experience* with various approaches, and the relative *risk–benefit* ratio. The following chapters cover those conditions, which we believe are best served by combination therapy based on the existing research and clinical experience:

■ Chapter 2: Major Depression
■ Chapter 3: Obsessive Compulsive Disorder
■ Chapter 4: Panic Disorder
■ Chapter 5: Posttraumatic Stress Disorder
■ Chapter 6: Sleep Disorders
■ Chapter 7: Schizophrenia
■ Chapter 8: Bipolar Disorder
■ Chapter 9: Borderline Personality
■ Chapter 10: Generalized Anxiety Disorder
■ Chapter 11: Conclusion

Each chapter includes an illustrative case presentation, which serves as an example in the discussion of diagnosis and treatment strategies. The case presentations are a compilation of numerous patient interactions chosen to best demonstrate the relevant issues.

TREATMENT ADHERENCE

A critical consideration relevant to this discussion is the issue of treatment adherence (or more accurately nonadherence) as a major potential obstacle to a successful outcome.[3] In this context, it is important to recognize that nonadherence is common and the degree to which it is present (i.e., as a continuum from total adherence to total nonadherence). Next, barriers to adequate adherence should be identified and addressed. Finally, a monitoring system acceptable to patients should be in place.

In general, the longer, the more expensive, and the more complicated a treatment strategy, the less likely a patient will (or can) adhere. Conversely, an approach that achieves a rapid resolution of symptoms may increase adherence. In this context, several issues should be considered when employing combined treatments, including:

- Patient's *access and acceptance* of specific forms of therapy
- The *affordability* in terms of time and money of various approaches
- The *available professional expertise* to properly administer specific treatments
- The *urgency* to ameliorate more disabling symptoms

Other factors that are often present and may undermine specific treatment strategies and decrease adherence include:

- *Comorbid psychiatric or medical* disorders
- *Comorbid alcohol and/or substance* use disorders
- Disorders at the *extremes of the age continuum* (e.g., pediatric depression, dementia with psychosis)

It is also important to consider whether the delivery of each approach is done by separate clinicians.[4] Such a scenario may compromise the successful integration of treatment and perpetuate a less effective dualistic model, essentially separating pharmacotherapy and psychotherapy. Gabbard[5] proposes ways to minimize this problem, emphasizing maintenance of open communication between prescriber and therapist (with the patient's informed consent) to address issues such as:

- *Emergencies*
- Treatment *changes*
- Treatment *termination*
- Differences in treatment *philosophies*

In summary, treatment adherence is critical to achieving an optimal outcome but is frequently compromised. Contributory factors can be illness related, treatment related, or patient related (see Table 1-1). Therefore, adequate monitoring and strategies to improve adherence are prerequisites to maximize the efficacy of any approach.

TABLE 1-1	*Factors That Contribute to Treatment Nonadherence*	
Illness Related	*Treatment Related*	*Patient Related*
Diagnosis	Efficacy	Acceptance of diagnosis and treatment
Illness and treatment duration	Tolerability	Stigma
Severity of symptoms	Safety	Inadequate social, economic support
History of poor adherence	Poor therapeutic relationship	Substance abuse
Severe depression		
Poor insight		
Cognitive impairment		

(Adapted from Lacro JP, Dunn LB, Dolder CR, et al. Prevalence of and risk factors for medication nonadherence in patients with schizophrenia: A comprehensive review of recent literature. *J Clin Psychiatry*. 2002;63(10):892–909.)[6]

TREATMENT STRATEGIES

Many treatment strategies assume that a psychotherapeutic approach (e.g., supportive, crisis intervention) is a preferable first step, particularly from a risk–benefit ratio. Several issues, however, may require initial medication intervention (alone or in combination with psychotherapy) if acute symptoms substantially impair the ability to function in important daily activities (e.g., work); represent an emergency (e.g., suicidal); or medication is the only viable approach (e.g., lack of access to or resources for the appropriate psychotherapy).

If psychotherapy is a viable first step but insufficient, then the next approach may involve switching to medication or adding medication. Conversely, if medication is the initial but inadequate first step then combining it with psychotherapy may be appropriate rather than switching to an alternative drug or drug combination. This also raises the issue of whether a combination strategy from the beginning of treatment or sequencing the two approaches (e.g., medication first to control symptoms sufficiently, then allowing patient's productive participation in psychotherapy) is the best option to maximize benefit while minimizing costs. When acute symptoms are stabilized, the next step involves the prevention of relapse (i.e., the continuation phase). Typically, this will involve persisting with the acute strategy found effective (i.e., medication or psychotherapy alone or their combination) for a sufficient period to assure stabilization. Once achieved, the next decision is whether to end treatment or incorporate "booster sessions" and how best to accomplish this. In disorders that have a high risk of recurrence, however, the appropriate approach is usually to develop an ongoing strategy (i.e., prophylaxis) to prevent (or at least minimize) the frequency and severity of future exacerbations. In each scenario, emphasis should be on utilizing the minimally effective approach including:

- A *gradual tapering of medication or psychotherapy*
- A *gradual tapering of either* approach when combined. The choice depends on issues such as the existing evidence base, a patient's tolerance to treatment, and the practicality of one approach versus the other
- *Maintenance of both* approaches at their minimally effective level

Another issue in this context is the type of psychotherapeutic approach that accomplishes the treatment goals in the most effective and efficient manner.[7] Therefore, psychotherapy may range from:

- Individual or family *supportive* sessions
- *Psychoeducational* approaches
- *Group, family,* or *marital* therapy
- Individual, group, online, or telephone *cognitive behavioral therapy*

In each chapter, we provide a treatment strategy that incorporates the integrated use of medication and psychotherapy as dictated by the evidence base for a specific disorder, level of symptom severity and chronicity, urgency to ameliorate symptoms, and the relative risk–benefit ratio of each step. A model for these strategies is provided in Figure 1-1.

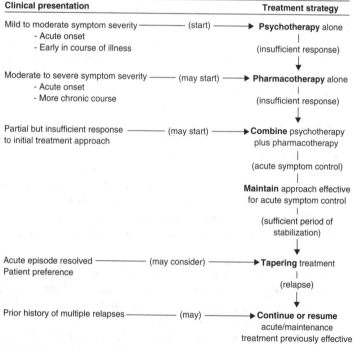

FIGURE 1-1 ■ Model treatment strategy integrating psychotherapy and pharmacotherapy.

REFERENCES

1. Gabbard GO. A neurobiologically informed perspective on psychotherapy. *Br J Psychiatry.* 2000;177:117–122.
2. Hollon SD, Fawcett J. Combined medication and psychotherapy for mood disorders. In: Gabbard GO, ed. *Gabbard's treatments of DSM-IV TR psychiatric disorders,* 4th ed. Arlington: American Psychiatric Press; 2007.
3. Osterberg L, Blaschke T. Adherence to medication. *N Engl J Med.* 2005;353(5):487–497.
4. Riba MB, Balon R. *Competency in combining pharmacotherapy and psychotherapy: integrated and split treatment,* 1st ed. Washington, DC: American Psychiatric Press; 2005.
5. Gabbard GO. The rationale for combining medication and psychotherapy. *Psychiatr Ann.* 2006;36(5):315–319.
6. Lacro JP, Dunn LB, Dolder CR, et al. Prevalence of and risk factors for medication nonadherence in patients with schizophrenia: A comprehensive review of recent literature. *J Clin Psychiatry.* 2002;63(10): 892–909.
7. Fisher JR, O'Donohue WT, eds. *Practitioner's guide to evidence-based psychotherapy.* New York: Springer; 2006.

SUGGESTED READINGS

Janicak PG, Davis JM, Preskorn SH, et al. *Principles and practice of psychopharmacotherapy,* 4th ed. Philadelphia: Lippincott Williams & Wilkins; 2006.
Kane JM. Review of treatments that can ameliorate nonadherence in patients with schizophrenia. *J Clin Psychiatry.* 2006;67(Suppl 5): 9–14.

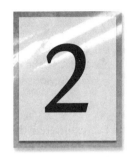

Major Depression

LEARNING OBJECTIVES

The reader will be able to:

1. Understand the differences and relationship between pharmacotherapy, device-based therapies, and psychotherapy for the treatment of major depression.
2. Develop strategies for combined or sequenced treatment approaches for major depression.
3. Enhance skills to negotiate these treatment approaches with patients.

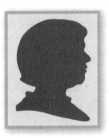

Ms. W

Ms. W is a 47-year-old, married woman with two adolescent children. She presented with symptoms of depressed mood, loss of interest and pleasure, poor concentration, hypersomnia, feelings of worthlessness, and inappropriate guilt. Ms. W denied symptoms of hypomania/mania in the past or currently. Screening with the Mood Disorders Questionnaire (MDQ) for bipolar disorder was negative. Her symptoms met diagnostic criteria for major depression. She has experienced three prior episodes since her late 20s with a full recovery between episodes. The current episode began 6 weeks ago. She initially refused medication because she did not like the side effects she experienced while on previous trials of antidepressants (ADs).

It is estimated that up to 14 million US adults will suffer from a major depression in any given year.[1] The American Psychiatric Association estimates the lifetime risk for experiencing a major depressive episode is 10% to 25% for women and 5% to 12% for men. This disorder is three times more likely to occur if an individual has a first-degree relative with depression. The risk is two to three times higher in females than males but this gap may be narrowing more recently with a higher number of young males experiencing depression. Depressive disorders are prevalent, debilitating, pose a higher risk for suicide, are associated with an increased risk of medical (e.g., cardiac) and other psychiatric (e.g., anxiety-related disorders) comorbidities, and are prone to recurrence. Further, a substantial proportion of individuals are insufficiently responsive to standard therapeutic approaches. Clinically meaningful levels of depression can occur in a variety of disorders, including:

- *Major depressive disorder* (single or recurrent, with or without melancholia, with or without psychosis, seasonal pattern)
- *Bipolar disorder* (depressed or mixed episodes)
- *Dysthymic disorder* (less severe, more chronic depressive symptoms)
- *Cyclothymic disorder* (fluctuation between dysthymic and hypomanic episodes)
- *Other psychiatric disorders* (e.g., schizoaffective disorder, depressed type)
- *Secondary to a general medical condition* (e.g., dementia with depression)
- *Substance-induced* mood disorder (e.g., stimulant withdrawal)

DIFFERENTIAL DIAGNOSIS

An important differential diagnosis involves *distinguishing unipolar major depression from bipolar disorder, depressed episode*. This may be difficult as the depressed phase of both disorders is similar and one or more depressions often precede the development of the characteristic hypomanic or manic episodes that define bipolar disorder. Nevertheless, it is critically important to clarify the diagnosis early in the course because treatment approaches are very different. The use of screening assessments such as the MDQ and the procurement of collateral sources of information can be helpful in this context (see Chapter 8). Another important differential issue is the *presence of psychotic symptoms*, which usually requires combining standard antidepressants (ADs) plus an antipsychotic. Finally, some patients experience recurrent depression that coincides with particular seasons. *Seasonal affective disorder* (SAD) often presents with atypical symptoms (e.g., hypersomnia, carbohydrate craving, and weight gain) and bright light therapy (BLT) may be effective (usually as an adjunct) for standard antidepressant treatments, particularly with the fall-onset pattern.

Regardless of the diagnosis, significant depressions usually involve disruption in mood, vegetative functions, and cognition (see Table 2-1). To meet diagnostic criteria, a major depressive episode should present with mood changes and associated vegetative and cognitive symptoms that persist for at least 2 weeks. Depression may be difficult to recognize given the myriad of presentations that occur across the life cycle. Table 2-2 lists some of the more common issues that characterize depression in various age-groups.

Ms. W reported that she was easily brought to tears, felt very tired, and was hopeless about the future. She was unable to work and only able to perform minimal daily activities related to the care of her children. At times, she was unable take a shower and once her children were in school, she would return to bed and sleep as much as she could. She denied suicidal ideation and had no history of attempts. Her symptoms had persisted for approximately 6 weeks.

Treatment-Resistant Depression

Treatment-resistant depression (TRD) is variably defined but a minimum criteria usually involves the persistence of significant depression despite two adequate treatment trials (e.g., two antidepressant trials, a cognitive behavioral therapy [CBT] trial and one

TABLE 2-1	*Symptoms of Depression*

Mood

- Depressed mood
- Diminished interest or pleasure (anhedonia)

Vegetative functions

- Weight or appetite change
- Sleep disturbance
- Psychomotor agitation or retardation
- Fatigue or loss of energy

Cognition

- Worthlessness/guilt/psychosis
- Diminished concentration or indecisiveness
- Hopelessness
- Suicidal ideation/intent/behavior

(Adapted from Janicak PG, Davis JM, Preskorn SH, et al. *Principles and practice of psychopharmacotherapy*, 4th ed. Philadelphia: Lippincott Williams & Wilkins; 2006.)

antidepressant trial). In this context, critical issues to consider are accuracy of diagnosis, adequacy of treatment (e.g., dose, number of sessions, duration), and patient adherence. On the basis of the results of the NIMH-sponsored Sequenced Treatment Alternatives to Relieve Depression (STAR*D) study, after two failed adequate trials the chances of achieving remission fall into the 10% to 20% range. Therefore, there is a significant need to develop more effective strategies in this population.

An important complication with unrecognized, inadequately treated, or persistent TRD is the increased *risk of suicide* which is the ninth leading cause of death in the United States for all ages and the third leading cause in adolescents and young adults. Depression contributes to 70% of suicides with a 15% mortality rate associated with untreated, recurrent major depression. Therefore, the need to assess for suicidal risk and to monitor carefully whenever a treatment intervention is initiated, altered, or stopped is paramount to prevent an otherwise

TABLE 2-2	*Common Issues that Characterize Depression in Different Age-Groups*

Prepubertal children

- Somatic complaints
- Agitation
- Anxiety
- Phobias

Adolescents

- Substance abuse
- Antisocial behavior
- Restlessness
- Truancy and other school difficulties
- Promiscuity
- Rejection hypersensitivity
- Poor hygiene

Adults

- Somatic complaints (particularly cardiovascular, gastrointestinal, genitourinary)
- Low back pain or other orthopedic symptoms

Elderly

- Cognitive deficits
- Pseudodementia
- Somatic complaints

(Adapted from Janicak PG, Davis JM, Preskorn SH, et al. *Principles and practice of psychopharmacotherapy*, 4th ed. Philadelphia: Lippincott Williams & Wilkins; 2006.)

unnecessary tragedy. While controversial, the U.S. Food and Drug Administration (FDA)-mandated black box warning for ADs to potentially increase suicidal ideation or behavior in pediatric, adolescent, and young adult populations does underscore the need to monitor these patients very carefully when these agents are prescribed.

NEUROBIOLOGY OF DEPRESSION

Our understanding of the neurobiology of depression is closely linked to the effects of various treatments (i.e., medications, psychotherapy, device-based treatments) on the central nervous system (CNS). Approaches to elucidating the mechanism subserving mood disorders involve multiple areas, including:

- *Genetic* risk is supported by *family, twin*, and *adoption studies*. Further, *interactions with the environment* and genetics appear critical to the development of depressive episodes. From another perspective, *pharmacogenetics* may soon help to predict chances of responding, dose requirements, and predilection to adverse effects (AEs).
- *Neuroanatomic* localization of *dysregulated neural circuits* is supported by imaging and postmortem studies.
- *Neurotransmitter systems* implicated in depression include the *serotonin, nonadrenergic,* and *dopaminergic* systems. *Other systems* also considered include the cholinergic, glutamatergic, γ-aminobutyric acid (GABA)ergic, histaminergic, and opioid systems.
- *Neuroendocrine system* may also play a role. For example, elevated *cortisol* levels due to dysregulation in the hypothalamic-pituitary axis (HPA) is an area of study regarding biomarkers for depression as well as novel treatment approaches (e.g., corticotropin-releasing hormone [CRH_1] antagonists).
- *Other hypotheses* involve disruption in *electrolytes* (e.g., K^+); *biological rhythms* (e.g., SAD; and the *immune system* (e.g., proinflammatory cytokines).

TREATMENT OF MAJOR DEPRESSION

Various treatment approaches or their combination have demonstrated benefit for depression. They include:

- *Pharmacotherapy*
  - ADs
  - Anxiolytics
  - Mood stabilizers
  - Antipsychotics (APs)

■ *Device-based therapy*
  ■ Electroconvulsive therapy (ECT)
  ■ Vagus nerve stimulation (VNS)
  ■ Possibly:
    □ Bright light therapy
    □ Transcranial magnetic stimulation (TMS)
    □ Deep brain stimulation (DBS)
■ *Psychotherapy*
  ■ CBT
  ■ Interpersonal psychotherapy (IPT)
  ■ Marital/family counseling
  ■ Group therapy

We will discuss each as a single approach and then explore the data to support their sequencing or combined use.

Pharmacotherapy for Major Depression

ADs can be divided into first- or second-generation agents (see Table 2-3) and further categorized by their putative mechanism of action (see Table 2-4).

On the basis of a balance between efficacy and safety/tolerability, the selective serotonin reuptake inhibitors (SSRIs) have become the first-line treatment approach for most patients. Factors that may dictate a specific SSRI or an alternate agent include a prior personal or family history of benefit to a certain antidepressant, susceptibility to certain AEs (e.g., sexual dysfunction), presence of comorbid psychiatric/medical disorders, potential for adverse drug interactions, and patient preference. Two critical issues to assure adequacy of an AD trial are the use of maximally tolerated doses (e.g., 40 mg of citalopram) for an adequate duration (e.g., 6 to 12 weeks). Increasingly, the goal is to achieve remission (i.e., minimal symptoms, good functioning) rather than response, usually defined as at least a 50% reduction in symptom severity. If adequacy and adherence are assured but benefit falls short of this target, then the next strategy involves switching to an alternate agent (within or out of class) particularly when response is absent to minimal. When there is a partial but insufficient response, an alternative approach is to augment the effect of the first treatment. This may involve combining medications or adding psychotherapy (e.g., CBT, IPT). In the context of the switching strategy, the results of the STAR*D study for

TABLE 2-3	*Medications for Treatment of Depression*

Class/Generic Name	Trade Name	Usual Daily Dosage (mg/d)
FIRST-GENERATION AGENTS		
TCA		
Amitriptyline	Elavil	75–300
Clomipramine	Anafranil	100–250
Desipramine	Norpramine	75–300
Doxepin	Sinequan	75–300
Imipramine	Tofranil	75–300
Nortriptyline	Pamelor	75–300
Protriptyline	Vivactil	20–60
Trimipramine	Surmontil	75–300
MAOI		
Isocarboxazid	Marplan	40–60
Phenelzine	Nardil	30–90
Selegiline[a]	Emsam	20 mg/20 cm^2 patch
Tranylcypromine	Parnate	30–60
SECOND-GENERATION AGENTS		
SSRI		
Citalopram	Celexa	20–40
Escitalopram	Lexapro	10–20
Fluoxetine	Prozac	10–60
Fluvoxamine[b]	Luvox	100–300
Paroxetine	Paxil	10–50
Sertraline	Zoloft	50–200
NRI		
Atomoxetine[b]		60–120
DSNRI		
Duloxetine	Cymbalta	30–60
Venlafaxine	Effexor	75–375
N-Desvenlafaxine	Pristiq	50–100

TABLE 2-3	*Medications for Treatment of Depression (continued)*	
Class/Generic Name	*Trade Name*	*Usual Daily Dosage (mg/d)*
Aminoketone		
Bupropion	Wellbutrin	150–450
Tetracyclic		
Amoxapine	Ascendin	200–600
Maprotiline	Ludiomil	75–225
Mirtazapine	Remeron	15–45
Triazolopyridine		
Nefazodone[c]	Serzone	100–600
Trazodone	Desyrel	150–600

[a]Transdermal system approved for depression.
[b]Not approved by the U.S. Food and Drug Administration for depression.
[c]Serzone no longer available; generic form of nefazodone still available.
SSRI, selective serotonin reuptake inhibitor; SNRI, selective norepinephrine reuptake inhibitor; DSNRI, dual serotonin norepinephrine reuptake inhibitor; TCA, tricyclic antidepressant; MAOI, monoamine oxidase inhibitor.
(Adapted from Janicak PG, Davis JM, Preskorn SH, et al. *Principles and practice of psychopharmacotherapy*, 4th ed. Philadelphia: Lippincott Williams & Wilkins; 2006.)

unipolar major depression indicate that an alternate SSRI (i.e., sertraline), an agent working through the catecholamine system (i.e., bupropion sustained release [SR]), a dual-acting agent (i.e., both serotonin and norepinephrine [NE] reuptake blockade [i.e., venlafaxine XR]), or CBT all produce similar levels of remission. Alternatively, augmenting with bupropion SR, buspirone (i.e., 5-hydroxytryptamine $[HT]_{1A}$ agonist), or CBT were also equally effective.[2] Another strategy, recently supported by clinical trials and increasingly employed in practice, is the addition of lower doses of a second-generation antipsychotic (SGA) (e.g., aripiprazole, quetiapine, risperidone) to augment the primary AD even in the absence of psychotic symptoms. In this context, aripiprazole is the first agent to receive FDA approval as an add-on treatment for major depressive disorder.

TABLE 2-4	Major Classes of Antidepressants Defined by Putative Mechanism of Action

5-HT and NE reuptake inhibition

- Tricyclic antidepressants (TCAs)
- Venlafaxine
- Duloxetine

5-HT reuptake inhibition

- Serotonin selective reuptake inhibitors (SSRIs)

5-HT$_2$ receptor blockers and SE uptake inhibition

- Nefazodone

Alternate 5-HT and NE actions

- Mirtazapine

NE reuptake inhibition

- Atomoxetine

DA and NE reuptake inhibition

- Bupropion

Monoamine oxidase inhibitors (MAOIs)

- Phenelzine
- Tranylcypromine
- Selegiline TS

HT, hydroxytryptamine; NE, norepinephrine; DA, dopamine; TS, transdermal system.

If these steps fail to achieve adequate benefit, a variety of alternative agents and device-based treatments, as well as switching, combining, and augmenting approaches have been less well studied but frequently used in clinical practice. These may include:

- *Switching* strategies to agents such as *tricyclic antidepressants* (TCAs) (e.g., nortriptyline) or *monoamine oxidase inhibitors* (MAOIs) (e.g., selegiline transdermal system [TS])

- *Combining* strategies to manage associated symptoms such as *anxiety* (e.g., lorazepam) or *sleep* problems (e.g., zolpidem)
- *Augmenting* strategies including *lithium; buspirone, thyroid hormone, stimulants* (e.g., methylphenidate, modafanil), *combined ADs*, or *SGAs*
- *Nutraceutical (NT)* strategies (e.g., St. John's Wort; S-adenosyl methionine [SAMe]; omega-3 fatty acids; inositol)

Of note, the *MAOIs* are presently the only class of ADs that impact all three commonly implicated NTs (i.e., NE, 5-HT, dopamine [DA]) and atomoxetine (presently approved for attention deficit hyperactivity disorder [ADHD]) is the only available selective norepinephrine reuptake inhibitor (SNRI) agent.

If bipolar depression is the diagnosis, then *mood stabilizer* monotherapy (e.g., lithium, lamotrigine, quetiapine) is ideal but not always adequate, especially with more severe presentations. Alternate approaches include:

- Combining mood stabilizers (e.g., lithium plus lamotrigine)
- Adding an AD to the primary mood stabilizer (e.g., SSRI plus divalproex sodium [DVPX])
- Device-based therapies (e.g., ECT, VNS)

Caution in using ADs is warranted given the increased potential to switch patients into hypomania/mania, to destabilize the long-term course of illness or to reduce response to a standard mood stabilizer. In this context, psychotherapy combined with a mood stabilizer may be a safer choice (see Chapter 8).

Once acute stabilization has been achieved, it is necessary to continue treatment at the acute levels to prevent relapse over the following 6 to 12 months. On the basis of the severity of an episode, level of response, and history of recurrent depression, it is then necessary to determine whether ongoing prophylactic treatment is warranted. In this context, the use of medication, psychotherapy and possibly device-based treatments may all play important roles.

A critical consideration in choosing a specific pharmacotherapy is an agent's safety/tolerability profile. Table 2-5 lists some of the more common AEs across the various classes of ADs. In addition, some of these medications are associated with specific AEs or toxicity, such as:

- *TCAs* may produce *cardiac arrhythmias*, particularly with toxic plasma levels.

| TABLE 2-5 | Antidepressants: Adverse Effects |

Drugs	Sedation	Anticholinergic	Orthostatic Hypotension	Cardiac Effects
FIRST-GENERATION AGENTS				
Tricyclics				
Amitryptyline	High	High	Moderate	High
Clomipramine	High	High	Low	Moderate
Desipramine	Low	Low	Low	Moderate
Doxepin	High	Moderate	Moderate	Moderate
Imipramine	Moderate	Moderate	High	High
Maprotiline	Moderate	Moderate	Low	Moderate
Nortriptyline	Moderate	Moderate	Low	Moderate
Protriptyline	Low	Moderate	Low	Moderate
Trimipramine	High	High	Moderate	High
Monoamine oxidase inhibitors				
Phenelzine	Low	None	High	None
Tranylcypromine	High	Very low	Very Low	None
Selegiline TS	Low	Low	High	Low
SECOND-GENERATION AGENTS				
Selective serotonin reuptake inhibitors				
Fluoxetine	Low	None	None	None
Paroxetine	Low	None	None	None
Sertraline	Low	None	None	None
Dibenzoxapines				
Amoxapine	Low	Low	None	None
Serotonin and norepinephrine reuptake inhibitors				
Venlafaxine	Low	Very low	Very low	Low
Duloxetine	Low	Very low	Low	Low
Aminoketones				
Bupropion	None	Very low	Moderate	Low
Serotonin and norepinephrine actions				
Mirtazapine	Moderate	Low	Low	Low

TABLE 2-5	*Antidepressants: Adverse Effects (continued)*			
Drugs	**Sedation**	**Anticholinergic**	**Orthostatic Hypotension**	**Cardiac Effects**
Phenylpiperazines				
Trazodone	High	Low	Moderate	Low
Nefazodone	Low	Low	Low	Low

(Adapted from Ward M. Appendix B. In: Flaherty J, Davis JM, Janicak PG, eds. *Psychiatry: diagnosis and therapy*, 2nd ed. Norwalk: Appleton & Lange; 1995:493–494.)

- *MAOIs* may produce drug–food interactions (i.e., *hypertensive crisis*) or drug–drug interactions (i.e., *serotonin syndrome*).
- *SSRIs* and *SNRIs* may cause *gastrointestinal* disturbances; initial *anxiety/agitation*; increased *suicidal ideation/behavior* in younger populations; or *sexual problems* with longer exposures (i.e., several weeks).
- *Bupropion* may cause *seizures*, particularly in patients with eating disorders or prior history of seizures.
- *Nefazodone* may cause *hepatic* toxicity.

 Ms. W was reluctant to consider antidepressant medication during the present episode, particularly because of diminished interest in sexual activities she experienced with previous SSRIs.

Possible discussion points include
- *Depression itself may cause sexual difficulties.*
- *When related to AD treatment, this AE may be improved by reducing the dose when clinically feasible or adding another agent to counteract this problem (e.g., bupropion, sildenafil).*
- *Certain ADs are less likely to cause this problem (e.g., bupropion, mirtazapine) and may be effective alternatives to an SSRI.*

Therefore, the choice of pharmacotherapy must strike a balance between efficacy and safety, keeping in mind any personal or familial proclivities that could increase benefit or predispose to a specific adverse event.

Device-Based Therapies for Major Depression

Therapeutic neuromodulation involves the use of device-based treatments that alter the electrical activity of relevant neurocircuits implicated in major depression. Three examples that are presently available include:

- ECT
- VNS
- BLT

Other approaches which are presently investigational are *TMS, magnetic seizure therapy* (MST), and *DBS*. Given the substantial proportion of depressed patients who are insufficiently responsive or intolerant to existing treatments (i.e., medication, psychotherapy), these approaches are being developed as alternative treatments administered alone or combined with medication and/or psychotherapy.

Psychotherapy for Major Depression

The American Psychiatric Association Practice Guidelines for Major Depression (revised) notes that several important issues regarding psychotherapy for the treatment of major depression need to be addressed, including:

- What are the *relative efficacies* among various psychotherapies?
- *What aspects of specific psychotherapies are efficacious* and whether they are common across all effective treatments?
- What are the *indications* (e.g., subtypes of depressive disorders) for different psychotherapies?
- Can different psychotherapies be effectively used *concurrently or sequentially*?
- What are the *optimal frequencies* of various psychotherapies for acute, continuation, or maintenance treatment?

There are several empirically supported psychotherapies for the treatment of the depression, including:

- Cognitive behavioral therapy (CBT)

- Interpersonal psychotherapy (IPT)
- Behavior therapy (BT)

In addition, there are several psychotherapies that show promising results but need further research. Those include:

- Exercise
- Social problem solving therapy
- Brief dynamic therapy
- Behavioral marital/family
- Mindfulness-based cognitive therapy

The use of the term *CT* in the literature is complicated. Although CT has been operationally defined, there are slight differences in how its various interventions are implemented. Because CT uses both cognitive and behavioral techniques, the terms *CT* and *CBT* have been used interchangeably. For purposes of this chapter, we will utilize the term *CBT*.

More than 40 years ago, Aaron Beck introduced cognitive therapy (CT) for the treatment of depression. This novel intervention focused on structured protocols that facilitated the ability to test it in randomized controlled trials. As a result, it has become one of the most studied interventions for depression. For example, in the STAR*D study, CBT was utilized and found comparable to standard medications in producing remission of major depression.

In general, the cognitive model of depression focuses on the *interaction between thoughts, affect, and behavior*. Treatment examines the negative views and interpretations that are associated with depression. Patients frequently alter the information they receive from the world to reinforce their negative view of themselves, their abilities, and their sense of hope for the future. These biased ideas manifest in *automatic thoughts*, which are quick and frequently go unreflected. In turn, these negative, automatic thoughts influence mood and behavior. CBT reflects and examines negative thoughts to ensure that they are accurate and, if not, develops the tools to manage them if they should reoccur. Recently, mindfulness-based CT has been introduced and includes the cognitive strategy of focussing on thoughts without judging or suppressing them.

At a deeper level, the cognitive model proposes that patients develop a *core set of beliefs* early in life about themselves and the world that contribute to the likelihood of developing depression. For example, an early belief could develop in a child who learns to believe that he or she is never good enough. The model proposes that eventually, with the right combination of stressors, that belief may activate and result in the person viewing the world from the perspective of not being able to adequately cope. Those early beliefs contribute to distortions and negative views of the world, which result in more depression. The CBT model focuses on understanding and altering such long-held beliefs and their accompanying automatic thoughts.

CBT sessions are very structured and begin with a *medication check* and/or a *mood check* usually with objective scores on a self-report questionnaire like the Beck Depression Inventory (BDI-II) or a Likert scale of depressed mood (0 to 10). Following the mood check, the therapist inquires about the patient's perception of the previous session to maintain consistency and get feedback or reactions. *Setting the agenda* for the session is the next important step followed by *working through the agenda* and the accompanying goals of treatment. The *homework* from the previous session is reviewed and new homework is assigned for next session. The session ends with a summary and feedback. For more information on the application of CBT see *Cognitive Behavioral Therapy for clinicians*.[3]

Interpersonal psychotherapy (*IPT*) has also been studied for the treatment of depression. IPT was developed by Klerman, Weissman et al. and addresses *interpersonal, social*, and *cultural factors*. It is a time limited, very focused treatment that helps patients *understand the biological or medical causes of depression* and centers on the *resolution of recent stressors and interpersonal problems* in their life. The IPT therapist helps patients understand how life events can cause depression, and assists them with managing negative feelings and guides them with their interpersonal conflicts. In the initial sessions (1 through 3), a diagnostic evaluation, an assessment of current interpersonal conflicts, and a presentation of the model and treatment contract is completed. Sessions 4 through 9 concentrate on resolving identified problems. The therapist focuses on current mood state and conflicts that have occurred since the last session. *Communication analysis* is an IPT tool used to deconstruct interpersonal conflicts and help the patient gain perspective and learn new ways to communicate. Sessions 10 through 12 focus on reinforcing progress, beginning termination, and preparing for a possible relapse.

BT is based on *learning theories of reinforcement* that propose increasing the frequency and quality of pleasant activities will positively influence mood. These activities can include social skills training, relaxation, and increasing pleasurable activities. BT is also problem focused and psychoeducational. Specific problems are addressed and an understanding of the treatment rationale is very important.

Social problem-solving therapy is another brief intervention that focuses on linking the patients' symptoms to their current problems, clarifying the current issues, and solving those problems in a very structured format. This type of therapy can be taught to other health care professionals and has been used in a variety of settings (i.e., primary care, nursing homes).

Brief dynamic therapy is a rapid-paced, dynamic therapy that focuses on underlying neurotic conflicts, defenses, and problematic relationship patterns. It does not focus on the reduction of symptoms directly but uses the relationship with the therapist to examine the ingrained patterns and interpersonal style that is causing conflict. This intervention has been manualized in a case book that outlines the strategies.[4]

Moderate physical activity is effective for reducing the symptoms of depression. Although this is typically defined as 30 minutes or more on most days, benefits have been shown with as little as a 10-minute brisk walk. It is suggested that clinicians introduce the benefits of physical activity and encourage patients to begin slowly, especially if they are inactive or experiencing substantial vegetative symptoms. To help patients start exercising, you need to work with them to overcome any barriers; encourage support from family or friends; and help them establish realistic, achievable goals. The therapist then gradually encourages patients to increase the frequency and length of physical exercise with a variety of enjoyable activities.

Combined Psychotherapy and Pharmacotherapy for Major Depression

Several studies and a recent meta-analysis report the combination of psychotherapy (e.g., IPT, CBT, BT, brief dynamic therapy) plus pharmacotherapy is superior to treatment with either modality alone. Further, sequencing a course of CBT in patients with only a partial response to medication may prevent relapse. Therefore, CBT may be effective as a stand-alone maintenance approach when successful as an acute treatment, an effective continuation treatment in patients responsive to acute treatment with medication, and help prevent relapse when combined with medication for continuation or maintenance treatment. In addition, there is data to support IPT as an effective maintenance approach given once monthly in depressed females who achieved clinical remission with this modality during the acute episode.

Many early trials concluded that CBT was superior to ADs; however, they were criticized for their inadequate medication regimens. More recent, better-controlled studies usually find CBT equally efficacious to ADs. Two studies, however, found CBT less effective than ADs. Both studies were large, multicentered, randomized, placebo-controlled trials. The first was the National Institute of Mental Health-Treatment of Depression Collaborative Research Program (NIMH-TDCRP) which found lower rates of improvement with CBT. They concluded that interpersonal psychotherapy (IPT) and ADs were superior to CBT in patients with more severe depression. The authors later reported, however, that sites with more experienced CBT clinicians had equivalent response rates compared to medication. This led others to conclude that expertise with CBT is an important factor when treating more severely depressed populations.[5]

The second study is the NIMH-sponsored Treatment for Adolescents with Depression Study (TADS). This trial randomized 439 adolescents (ages 12 to 17) with major depression to one of four treatments over 12 weeks:

- Fluoxetine alone (10 to 40 mg/day)
- CBT alone
- CBT plus fluoxetine
- Placebo alone

The medication tablets (i.e., fluoxetine or placebo) were administered under double-blind conditions, whereas CBT alone or combined with fluoxetine was administered in an unblinded manner. The authors concluded that the combination of CBT and ADs was most effective, whereas CBT alone was no more effective than placebo. The appropriate application of CBT, however, was questioned by Weisz et al.[6] because effect sizes achieved with CBT were smaller than those in previous studies.

Subsequently, the long-term effectiveness and safety of these treatment strategies were assessed in an open-labeled design for up to 36 weeks. Of note, rates of response were comparable between the combined treatment (85%), fluoxetine alone (81%), and CBT alone (81%) at this time point. Further, suicidal events were less common in patients receiving combined treatment (8.4%) or CBT alone (6.3%) versus fluoxetine alone (14.7%).

Introducing Combined Treatment

 Ms. W presented with significant feelings of hopelessness. She denied any suicidal ideation but many patients do not share their intent. Her levels of hopelessness and low functioning were a cause of concern, so we began to discuss the idea of combined treatment early in her care. We discussed the likely benefits of combined treatment when she would describe vegetative symptoms like sleep disturbance, agitation, low energy, and poor concentration. It was also discussed that psychotherapy alone may be beneficial. The patient chose psychotherapy alone and treatment focused on cognitive and behavioral strategies. Owing to her severe feelings of hopelessness, however, the discussion also included how medication may help in addition to CBT.

Possible discussion points include
- *Depression can be overwhelming and make you feel like you cannot do anything right.*
- *Sometimes medication can take the edge off the symptoms you are experiencing.*
- *This may then help you use your coping skills.*
- *For example, the medication may help with your sleep or increase your energy so you can then try some positive things (e.g., exercising), which in turn may lift your mood for a few moments.*
- *Little by little those positive moments may last longer and longer.*

If one clinician is unable to provide both interventions, an important element of combined treatment is communication between providers. Treatment may be enhanced when both providers are communicating their progress and experiences with the patient. Following a discussion outlining confidentiality and its limits, patients should sign a release of information allowing the collaborating clinicians to exchange information. There are several important questions to consider for major depression which are as follows:

Questions to ask the psychotherapist
- What are the patient's treatment goals?
- What progress have you seen?
- Has the patient identified any suicidal ideation?
- How are the scores on the BDI-II?
- How can I help with treatment goals?

Questions to ask the pharmacotherapist
- What symptoms are you targeting?
- Has the patient identified any suicidal ideation?
- How long will you try this medication?
- Are you planning any adjustments?
- What symptom changes have you noted?

CLINICAL RECOMMENDATIONS

For the acute treatment of a major depressive episode (mild to moderate in severity), we would initiate treatment with a second-generation AD; an agent that was previously beneficial; or CBT or IPT based on the patient's preference and their availability. With marked agitation, anxiety or dysomnia, panic symptoms, or acute suicidality we would introduce temporary adjunctive anxiolytics/sedative hypnotics. For an acute severe depressive episode, we would initiate combined treatment with a second-generation AD and CBT or IPT.

With minimal to no response, we would switch to an alternate AD (preferably of a different class) or consider an MAOI if the clinical presentation is atypical. If partial response is achieved, we would consider augmenting with various medications including two ADs from different classes or CBT or IPT (if not used initially). Alternatively, we would consider an SGA, particularly if psychotic symptoms are present or response to previous interventions was insufficient. In patients who do not respond to the treatment mentioned in the preceding text, are acutely suicidal, have a history of poor response to medication or psychotherapy, or a good previous response to ECT, we would consider initiating a trial with ECT or perhaps TMS (if clinically available).

Alternative strategies for those patients where psychotherapy is not accessible include support groups, telephone treatment, online CBT and self-help books. Telephone treatments have been developed and appear to provide benefit. More recently, several studies have examined online or Internet CBT for patients experiencing mild to moderate depression. However, Spek et al.[7] in a meta-analysis of these studies, found only small effect sizes with significant heterogeneity which they attributed to the varied therapist support provided in the programs. In the future, online CBT may be an alternative especially for those with mild depression.

There are numerous self-help books published for depression, some that incorporate CBT techniques and strategies and have been shown effective. Those include the well-known *Feeling Good* series by Dr. Burns.[8] This series has been published in several formats (i.e., workbook) and is readily available at bookstores. In addition, Copeland et al.[9,10] and McQuaid and Carmona[11] have published several workbooks. Petit et al.[12] published a self-help book focusing on interpersonal issues for the treatment of depression. Those who are less familiar with CBT or IPT can review several available books to learn the techniques and interactions.[13,14]

To prevent relapse, we would continue the same strategy effective for the acute episode for 6 to 12 months after stabilization. With a history of frequent recurrence or reemergence of symptoms, we would use the effective acute strategy as indefinite maintenance treatment.

 Ms. W experienced a significant decrease in her depressive symptoms with CBT. Her mood and energy improved. Her functioning increased significantly with improved concentration and her hopelessness disappeared. She also consolidated her sleep with the addition of CBT for sleep disorders (see Chapter 5). Ms. W continued weekly CBT for 6 months. As her symptoms remained stable, we began to decrease the frequency of her sessions to every other week and eventually moved to a booster session model after 9 months.

Figures 2-1 and 2-2 outline the approaches we would recommend for acute and maintenance treatment of unipolar major depression.

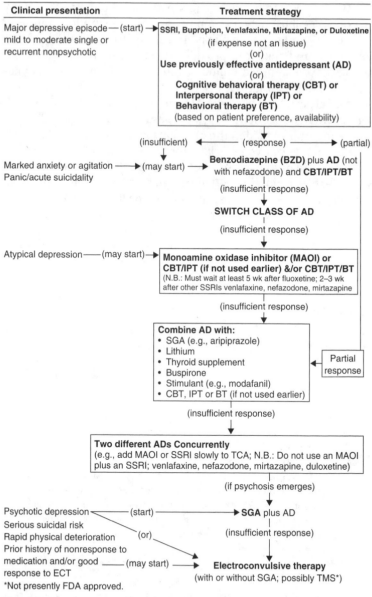

FIGURE 2-1 ■ Acute treatment strategy for major depressive episode. SSRI, selective serotonin reuptake inhibitor; AD, antidepressant; SGA, second-generation antipsychotic; TCA, tricyclic antidepressant; TMS, transcranial magnetic stimulation. (Adapted from Janicak PG, Davis JM, Preskorn SH, et al. *Principles and practice of psychopharmacotherapy*, 4th ed. Philadelphia: Lippincott Williams & Wilkins; 2006:254.)

Clinical presentation	Treatment strategy

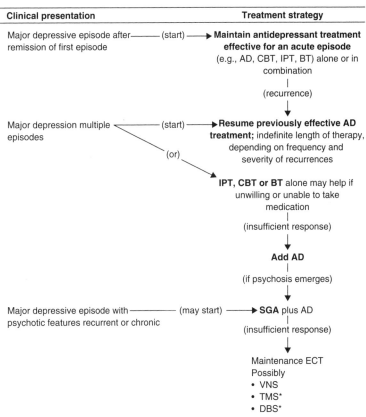

Major depressive episode after——— (start) ——→ **Maintain antidepressant treatment**
remission of first episode   **effective for an acute episode**
                                               (e.g., AD, CBT, IPT, BT) alone or in
                                                         combination

                                                       (recurrence)

Major depression multiple ———— (start) ——→ **Resume previously effective AD**
episodes   **treatment;** indefinite length of therapy,
                                                       depending on frequency and
                                        (or)   severity of recurrences

                                               IPT, CBT or BT alone may help if
                                               unwilling or unable to take
                                                         medication
                                                   (insufficient response)

                                                        Add AD

                                                   (if psychosis emerges)

Major depressive episode with ——————— (may start) ——→ **SGA** plus AD
psychotic features recurrent or chronic   (insufficient response)

                                                      Maintenance ECT
                                                      Possibly
                                                      • VNS
                                                      • TMS*
                                                      • DBS*

*Not presently FDA approved.

FIGURE 2-2 ▦ Maintenance strategy for recurrent depression.
AD, antidepressant; CBT, cognitive behavioral therapy; IPT, interpersonal
psychotherapy; BT, behavioral therapy; SGA, second-generation
antipsychotic; ECT, electroconvulsive therapy; VNS, vagus nerve stimulation;
TMS, transcranial magnetic stimulation; DBS, deep brain stimulation.
(Adapted from Janicak PG, Davis JM, Preskorn SH, et al. *Principles and practice
of psychopharmacotherapy*, 4th ed. Philadelphia: Lippincott Williams & Wilkins;
2006:260.)

Learning points

- Second-generation ADs (e.g., SSRIs, venlafaxine, bupropion) are the preferred pharmacotherapies for depression.
- CBT, BT, and interpersonal psychotherapy are the psychotherapeutic treatments of choice for depression.
- Combination strategies may enhance benefits in those unresponsive to either treatment approach alone.

REFERENCES

1. Kessler RC, Berglund P, Demler O, et al. The epidemiology of major depressive diorder: Results from the National Survey Replication (NCS-R). *JAMA*. 2003;289(23):3095–3105.
2. Gilmer WS, Kemp DE. STAR*D: What have we learned thus far? *Int Drug Ther Newsl*. 2006;41(10):75–82.
3. Sudak D. *Cognitive behavioral therapy for clinicians. Psychotherapy in clinical practice*. Lippincott Williams & Wilkins; 2006.
4. Levinson H. *Time-limited dynamic psychotherapy: a guide to clinical practice*. New York: Basic Books; 1995.
5. Hollon SD, Thase ME, Markowitz JC. Treatment and prevention of depression. *Psychol Sci Public Interest*. 2002;3:39–77.
6. Weisz JR, Weersing VR. Community clinic treatment of depressed youth: Benchmarking usual care against CBT clinicial trials. *J consult clin Psychol*. 2002;70(2):299–310.
7. Spek V, Cuijpers P, Nyklicek I, et al. Internet-based cognitive behavioral therapy for symptoms of depression and anxiety: A meta-analysis. *Psychol Med*. 2007;37(3):319–328.
8. Burns D. *Feeling good handbook*. New York: Plume; 1999.
9. Copeland ME. *The depression workbook: a guide for living with depression and manic depression*, 2nd ed. Oakland: New Harbinger Publications, Inc; 2001.
10. Copeland ME, Copans S. *Recovering from depression: a workbook for teens*. Baltimore: Paul H. Brookes Publishing; 2002.
11. McQuaid JR, Carmona PE. *Peaceful mind: using mindfulness and cognitive behavioral psychology to overcome depression*. New Harbinger Publications; 2004.
12. Pettit JW, Joiner TE, Rehm LP. *The interpersonal solution to depression: a workbook for changing how you feel by changing how you relate (New Harbinger self-help workbook)*. New Harbinger Publications; 2005.

13. Barlow DH. *Clinical handbook of psychological disorders.* New York: The Guilford Press; 2007:250–364.
14. Beck J. *Cognitive therapy.* New York: The Guilford Press; 1995.

SUGGESTED READINGS

American Psychiatric Association. Practice guideline for the treatment of patients with major depressive disorder (Revision). *Am J Psychiatry.* 2000;157(Suppl 4):1–45.

Beck AT, Ward CH, Mendelson M, et al. An inventory of measuring depression. *Arch Gen Psychiatry.* 1961;4:53–63.

Byrne NA, Regan CB, Livingston GB. Adherence to treatment in mood disorders. *Curr Opin Psychiatry.* 2006;19(10):44–49.

Fisher JR, O'Donohue WT, eds. *Practitioner's guide to evidence-based psychotherapy.* New York, NY: Springer; 2006.

Frank E, Kupfer DJ, Buysse DJ, et al. Randomized trial of weekly, twice-monthly, and monthly interpersonal psychotherapy as maintenance treatment for women with recurrent depression. *Am J Psychiatry.* 2007;164(5):761–767.

Friedman MA, Detweiler-Bedell JB, Leventhal HE, et al. Combined psychotherapy and pharmacotherapy for the treatment of major depressive disorder. *J Clin Psychol: Sci Pract.* 2004;11:47–68.

Goldapple K, Segal Z, Garson C, et al. Modulation of cortical-limbic pathways in major depression: Treatment-specific effects of cognitive behavior therapy. *Arch Gen Psychiatry.* 2004;61(1):34–41.

Hirschfeld RM, Calabrese JR, Weissman MM, et al. Screening for bipolar disorder in the community. *J Clin Psychiatry.* 2003;64(1):53–59.

Hollon SD, Jarrett RB, Nierenberg AA, et al. Psychotherapy and medication in the treatment of adult and geriatric depression: which monotherapy or combined treatment. *J Clin Psychiatry.* 2005;66(4):455–468.

Janicak PG, Davis JM, Preskorn SH, et al. *Principles and practice of psychopharmacotherapy,* 4th ed. Philadelphia: Lippincott Williams & Wilkins; 2006.

Janicak PG, Dowd SM, Martis B, et al. Repetitive transcranial magnetic stimulation versus electroconvulsive therapy for major depressive: preliminary results of a randomized trial. *Biol Psychiatry.* 2002;51:659–667.

Jarrett RB, Kraft D, Doyle J, et al. Preventing recurrent depression using cognitive therapy with and without a continuation phase: a randomized clinical trial. *Arch Gen Psychiatry.* 2001;58(4):381–388.

de Jonghe F, Hendricksen M, van Aalst G, et al. Psychotherapy alone and combined with pharmacotherapy in the treatment of depression. *Br J Psychiatry.* 2004;185:37–45.

Keller MB, McCullough JP, Klein DN, et al. A comparison of nefazodone, the cognitive behavioral-analysis system of psychotherapy, and their combination for the treatment of chronic depression. *N Engl J Med.* 2000;342(20):1462–1470.

Khurshid K, Janicak PG. Transcranial magnetic stimulation for the treatment of neuropsychiatric disorders other than depression. *Psychiatr Ann.* 2005;35(2):146–158.

March J, Silva S, Petrycki S, et al. Treatment for adolescents with depression study (TADS) team. Fluoxetine, cognitive behavioral therapy, and their combination for adolescents with depression: Treatment for Adolescents with Depression Study (TADS) randomized controlled trial. *JAMA.* 2004;292(7):807–820.

March JS, Silva S, Petrycki S, et al. The Treatment for Adolescents with Depression Study (TADS): long-term effectiveness and safety outcomes. *Arch Gen Psychiatry.* 2007;64(10):1132–1144.

Pampallona S, Bollini P, Tibaldi G, et al. Combined pharmacotherapy and psychological treatment for depression: A systematic review. *Arch Gen Psychiatry.* 2004;61(7):714–719.

Thase ME, Greenhouse JB, Frank E, et al. Treatment of major depression with psychotherapy or psychotherapy-pharmacotherapy combinations. *Arch Gen Psychiatry.* 1997;54(11):1009–1015.

Weisz JR, MacCarty CA, Valeri SM. Effects of psychotherapy for depression in children and adolescents: A meta-analysis. *Psychol Bull.* 2002;132:132–149.

3

Obsessive Compulsive Disorder

LEARNING OBJECTIVES

The reader will be able to:

1. Understand the differences and relationship between pharmacotherapy and psychotherapy for the treatment of obsessive compulsive disorder (OCD).
2. Develop strategies for combined or sequenced treatment approaches for OCD.
3. Enhance skills to negotiate these treatment approaches with patients.

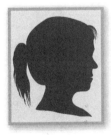

Ms. V

Ms. V is a 28-year-old, single female, living with her parents and 9-year-old child. she presented with an intense fear of contamination combined with multiple rituals that interfered with her functioning and met diagnostic criteria for obsessive compulsive disorder (OCD). Although treated with fluvoxamine (250 mg per day), she continued to experience significant anxiety and compulsive behaviors and her psychiatrist referred her for integrated treatment. Ms. V has been treated for the last 10 years after being hospitalized at age 18 because her anxiety and ritual behaviors were overwhelming. At the initial psychological evaluation she stated that she "did not want to touch a toilet." In the past, she typically stopped attending individual therapy sessions after a few months.

According to the National Institute of Mental Health (NIMH) Epidemiologic Catchment Area Study, the lifetime prevalence of OCD is approximately 2.5%. Onset occurs before age 21 in 50% of patients and symptoms fluctuate in severity but typically persist throughout life. Psychological problems postulated to underlie OCD include an abnormality in risk assessment, pathological doubt, and the need for certainty or perfection.

OCD consists of *obsessions* (i.e., persistent ideas, thoughts, impulses, or images) that originate internally and are perceived as intrusive and senseless. Typical themes include:

- Contamination
- Aggression
- Safety or harm
- Sex
- Religious scruples
- Physical concerns
- Need for symmetry or exactness

To neutralize these experiences, *compulsive behaviors* are performed usually in a stereotypical manner as per a set of rules. Typical behaviors include:

- Cleaning
- Washing
- Checking
- Excessive ordering and arranging
- Counting
- Repeating
- Collecting

In addition, *hoarding* may represent a distinct OCD subtype.[1,2] For example, there is genetic data to support biological differences between patients having OCD with or without hoarding.[3,4] Further, these patients may have a more severe form of the illness (e.g., poorer insight, greater indecisiveness, greater prevalence of social phobia, and generalized anxiety disorder, more severe compulsions, greater impairment, and dysphoria). Finally, although some data indicate a poorer response to treatment, this is yet to be adequately resolved.[5]

To meet diagnostic levels, these experiences should cause distress, consume significant time, and interfere with normal daily activities. Presently, there is ongoing debate as to the classification of OCD as separate from other anxiety disorders.

Ms. V experienced intense fears of being contaminated which caused her to conduct several washing rituals in the shower. Many times her showers took >2 hours. Throughout the day she continued to fear contamination, was careful about what she touched and where she sat, and washed her hands repeatedly throughout the day. Sometimes she required her family's assistance in child care when unable to withstand the anxiety about being dirty.

DIFFERENTIAL DIAGNOSIS

Comorbid conditions are frequent with as many as 50% of patients with OCD also experiencing a major depression. Phobias, panic disorder, and alcohol abuse are also more frequent with OCD in comparison with the general population. The strong association with *Gilles de la Tourette syndrome* is notable given the likely genetic basis of this condition. Finally, a variety of conditions manifest symptoms that are reminiscent of OCD, have familial patterns, and often respond to similar treatments. These include:

- Body dysmorphic disorder
- Trichotillomania
- Tic disorders
- Hypochondriasis
- Obsessive compulsive personality disorder

This has given rise to the concept of obsessive compulsive spectrum disorder (OCSD).

NEUROBIOLOGY OF OBSESSIVE COMPULSIVE DISORDER

The biology of OCD has been considered from several perspectives including:

- *Familial/genetic* studies that find a higher prevalence in first-degree relatives
- *Imaging* studies that implicate the anterior cingulate-basal ganglia-thalamocortical circuit
  - For example, *basal ganglia dysfunction* often manifests OCD symptoms (e.g., Huntington disease)
- *Neurotransmitter* dysregulation (e.g., 5-hydoxytryptamine [5-HT] transporter, Dopamine [DA] receptor type 4, glutamate transporter, γ-aminobutyric acid [GABA] type B receptor 1)

TREATMENT OF OBSESSIVE COMPULSIVE DISORDER

Both pharmacotherapy and psychotherapy have demonstrated efficacy in the management of OCD. The choice of either approach or their combination is dictated by such factors as:

- Level of *insight*
- Symptom *severity*
- Level of *disability*
- *Good prior response* to a specific approach
- *Level of response* to initial monotherapy
- *Chronicity*
- *Comorbid* disorders
- Patient *preference*
- Treatment *availability*

We first describe the evidence to support each approach as a monotherapy and then discuss their sequencing and combination. In this context, data suggest that the combination of therapies is more effective in some but not all patients.

Pharmacotherapy for Obsessive Compulsive Disorder

The preponderance of evidence supports the role of agents that block 5-HT reuptake into presynaptic neurons.[6] In this context, an important observation is the unique benefit of clomipramine in comparison to other tricyclic antidepressants (TCAs) and monoamine oxidase inhibitors (MAOIs).[7] Although this agent involves both NE and 5-HT reuptake inhibition, it is singularly more potent in its 5-HT actions relative to other agents in its class. This action, coupled with the known efficacy of selective serotonin reuptake inhibitors (SSRIs) for OCD, identifies this neurotransmitter as a critical target for therapeutic effects. Although earlier data supported a preferential benefit for clomipramine over other SSRIs, subsequent comparison trials have not proved the same.[8] Given the more significant adverse effects and similar efficacy of clomipramine, an SSRI is the recommended first-line medication approach. Although not all SSRIs have a U.S. Food and Drug Administration (FDA)-approved indication for OCD, it is likely that they all would be effective. An adequate trial may involve higher doses (e.g., sertraline 400 mg per day) for a more extended duration (e.g., 12 weeks). An unsuccessful or partially beneficial trial dictates trying another SSRI because there is ample evidence that insufficient response to one agent in class does not mean that a second SSRI would also fail. Choice of specific SSRIs should be guided by factors such as:

- *Prior history* of responsiveness
- Presence of *comorbid* psychiatric and/or medical disorders
- *Safety/tolerability* profile
- Potential for *drug interactions*

Dose titration schedules may require a conservative (i.e., lower doses, less frequent increments) approach to insure tolerability and the ultimate achievement of an adequate trial. The downside of this approach is the more extended time frame to achieve adequate treatment levels (see Table 3-1).

TABLE 3-1	Medications for Treatment of Obsessive Compulsive Disorder (OCD)[9]		
Class/Generic Name	Common Trade Name	Usual Drug Dosage (mg/d)	Usual Maximum Dose (mg/d)
SSRIs			
[a]Citalopram	Celexa	40–60	80
[a]Escitalopram	Lexapro	20	40
Fluoxetine	Prozac	40–60	80
Fluvoxamine	Luvox	200	300
Paroxetine	Paxil	40–60	60
Sertraline	Zoloft	200	200
TCAs			
Clomipramine	Anafranil	100–250	250

[a]Not FDA approved for OCD.
SSRI, selective serotonin reuptake inhibitor; TCA, tricyclic antidepressant.
(Adapted from Koran LM, Hanna GL, Hollander E, et al. Practice guideline for the treatment of patients with obsessive-compulsive disorder. *Am J Psychiatry*. 2007;164[Suppl 7]:22.)

If adequate symptom control remains elusive, adding psychotherapy or switching to clomipramine is indicated. The combined approach is discussed later in this chapter. As noted earlier, the potential efficacy of clomipramine is muted by its adverse effect profile, which is similar to other TCAs. These include:

- *Anticholinergic* effects (e.g., dry mouth, constipation, cognitive effects)
- *Antihistaminic* effects (e.g., sedation, weight gain)
- *α-Adrenergic* effects (e.g., hypotension)
- *Sodium channel* effects (e.g., cardiac rhythm disturbance)

Starting at low doses ($\leq$25 mg per day) and gradually titrating up may allow for acclimation to these effects in many patients.

With lack of adequate response after the steps mentioned earlier, the evidence base is much less robust in dictating the next strategies. Pharmacologic approaches include selective serotonin and norepinephrine reuptake inhibitors (SNRIs) such as venlafaxine, mirtazapine; SSRI augmentation with one or more trials of different first-generation antipsychotics (FGAs) or second-generation antipsychotics (SGAs); or buspirone.

Discontinuing successful acute treatment is a complicated decision. Most experts agree that a minimum maintenance period of 1 to 2 years should elapse before considering a cessation of therapy. Relapse rates and time to relapse in discontinuation trials vary widely but generally indicate that a substantial number of patients will experience a recurrence. Therefore, indefinite pharmacotherapy should be considered in all patients. If attempted, tapering of treatment should be slow (i.e., 10% to 25% decrease monthly) with careful monitoring for symptom worsening.

Device-Based Therapies for Obsessive Compulsive Disorder

In more severe unremitting courses, device-based, neuromodulatory therapies and psychoses general procedures have been studied or utilized, including the following:

- Neurosurgery
  - Anterior capsulotomy
  - Limbic leukotomy
  - Cingulotomy
  - Gamma-knife radiosurgery
- Deep brain stimulation (DBS)
- Transcranial magnetic stimulation (TMS)

Psychotherapy for Obsessive Compulsive Disorder

OCD is a complicated illness with a high rate of treatment avoidance. It is estimated that up to 30% of patients who initiate psychotherapy drop out of treatment.[10] The only empirically supported psychotherapeutic treatment for OCD is cognitive behavioral therapy (CBT). There are currently no studies examining the success of other psychotherapeutic interventions (e.g., psychodynamic, interpersonal).

The development of psychotherapy for OCD illustrates the evolution of psychotherapy in general. The early treatments in this specialty concentrated on psychodynamic interpretations but were not very successful. In the late 1960s the focus on behavioral interventions and learning theory formed a new psychotherapeutic paradigm. Over time, criticisms of behaviorism and its possible limitations led to a focus on cognitive interventions. The treatment for OCD has mirrored that evolution. Exposure and response prevention (ERP) became the treatment of choice because this behavioral model was very successful. Many patients, however, did not respond or could not tolerate ERP. As a result, cognitive therapy (CT) techniques were then used to treat OCD due to their success with other anxiety disorders. CT focuses less on exposure and more on cognitive restructuring. In our estimation the distinction is subtle. In this chapter, the terms *ERP* and *CBT* are used interchangeably and emphasize the behavioral intervention component.

As noted earlier, CBT is a treatment approach focused on current symptoms and based on learning theories. In general, the CBT therapist examines maladaptive thoughts that influence mood and behavior. CBT typically incorporates cognitive and behavioral aspects with the focus on either of those components dependent on the presenting symptoms and clinician preference. Research examining which of those two components (i.e., cognitive, behavioral) is most efficacious is difficult to interpret and the results are varied. As with other disorders, the primary effective treatment component of CBT for OCD is debated. For further information on the application of CBT, see *Cognitive Behavioral Therapy for clinicians*.[11]

What is clear is that ERP is considered the treatment of choice for OCD. ERP involves a prolonged and paced approach of exposure to obsessional cues or thoughts combined with an attempt to restrict any compensatory rituals. These exposures occur either with the use of imagery or in real-life settings (*in vivo*). The use of imagery or *in vivo* exposure depends on the feared situation. Many unrealistic fears cannot be recreated *in vivo* but require the patient to imagine them. In ERP, patients expose themselves to the causes of their obsessional fear and are required to stay in that situation while refraining from any rituals or avoidance until the distress decreases.

The use of ERP was first described in 1966 by Meyer.[12] It developed from the theory that repeated exposure to feared thoughts or situations habituates the person to anxiety and helps them disconnect the anxiety or fear from the ritual. As a result, they no longer need the rituals because the potential disaster or feared results do not occur during the exposures. Naturally, this approach runs completely counter to the patient's coping skills and can be very challenging. Therefore, ERP typically begins with moderately difficult situations, and while matching the patient's level of comfort, proceeds until the most distressing situations are faced. The patient completes the exposures in session and practices self-exposure at home between sessions.

A typical ERP session includes ranking the feared stimulus on a scale of 1 to 100 (Subjective Units of Distress Scale or SUDS). The plan is to generate a list of 10 to 15 items with varying degrees of anxiety associated with each task. In addition, time is spent collecting information regarding the rituals and the avoidance of fears. Homework may be assigned to gather information that can help with the treatment planning. In the present case, the patient kept a log of her washing rituals.

Using the information gathered, the patient and therapist collaboratively establish a treatment plan in which the patient gradually exposes himself or herself to the lower-rated fears. For patients afraid of contamination, this may include touching the light switch or the bottom of their shoe. Once all the information about the habit has been gathered, there is a commitment from the patient and a plan has been established, exposure begins. By the second or third session, an item on the hierarchy is chosen for the first exposure. At a rate of approximately every 10 to 15 minutes during the exposure, the therapist checks for a SUDS rating. It is important to remain focused on the feared contamination and not distract from the exposure during this time. Once the anxiety is significantly decreased, as measured by self-report and SUDS ratings, the session is completed and homework assigned to continue the contamination in some form. This may include contaminating an object that the patient will carry in their pocket.

 Ms. V was introduced to ERP in the past as she noted at the initial evaluation when she expressed her fears of having to "touch a toilet." She described complete dread over the idea of exposing herself to contamination. Her situation clearly illustrated the need for combined treatment, with medication reducing her symptoms sufficiently to allow consideration of the challenges inherent in ERP. In collaboration with the patient, the target situations that caused mild to moderate distress were established and gradually, as the patient was successful, she stepped up the hierarchy to those situations with higher distress.

Recent evidence suggests that CT may be as effective as ERP. CT involves shorter exposures with more focus on cognitive restructuring or challenging the dysfunctional thoughts that underlie the obsessional fear. CT emphasizes that intrusive thoughts are normal and it is the patient's interpretation of those thoughts that is distressing. CT focuses on understanding the randomness of thoughts, correcting erroneous beliefs, and testing out certain fears. Clinicians who utilize ERP, however, argue that it leads to cognitive adaptation and that the differences in these treatments are at best subtle. In this context, ERP and CT were directly compared and found equally effective.[13] More recently, these two interventions have been combined. At this point, however, ERP is considered to be the first-line treatment with a more cognitive approach employed if there are comorbid illnesses or ERP alone is insufficient.

Combined Psychotherapy and Pharmacotherapy for Obsessive Compulsive Disorder

In the reality of clinical practice, most patients receive combined treatment. In this context, psychotherapy can take many forms including individual, family, or group. The largest database, however, supports CBT or ERP as the most effective approaches.

There are also trials examining the combined efficacy of ERP and medication. Cottraux[14] compared ERP, fluvoxamine, and their combination and found the combined treatment more effective at the end of the acute phase but this benefit did not persist at 6 months follow-up. O'Connor et al.[15] included 29 subjects with OCD who were randomized to the following modes of treatment:

- Medication and CBT
- CBT only

- Medication and wait list for CBT
- No medication and wait list for CBT

They reported that all groups significantly improved except those on the "No medication and CBT wait list." Although the authors concluded that the combined treatment further enhanced efficacy, they felt it is more clinically beneficial to introduce CBT after a period of medication rather than initiating both treatments together. In a later trial involving 43 subjects with OCD, O'Connor et al.[16] reported that CBT alone was comparable in efficacy to CBT plus fluvoxamine. They noted, however, that while CBT successfully reduced obsessions, combined treatment produced a greater improvement in mood.

Introducing Combined Treatment

 Ms. V, while experiencing a mild reduction in compulsive behaviors after starting fluvoxamine, still spent significant time with washing rituals. Because she continued to struggle with her illness, her psychiatrist took this opportunity to open up the discussion about combining treatments.

Possible discussion points include:

- *In my experience, obsessions and compulsions can be very powerful. Sometimes, the anxiety is so overwhelming you cannot imagine how you are going to make it.*
- *Medications are very helpful in reducing your anxiety and physical tension but sometimes we need additional tools or strategies to help cope.*
- *I want to talk to you about CBT. This is a type of treatment that can help some people.*
- *CBT works by helping you to look at your fears and learn new ways to cope with them.*
- *I would like you to think about whether you are ready to learn some new tools to help your OCD.*

Following the initial introduction and once a patient begins to consider the option to pursue CBT, it is very important to clearly describe the treatment before referral. Owing to the nature of ERP, many patients will refuse treatment because the thought of exposing themselves to their fears is overwhelming. Therefore, it is important to help the patient complete a cost–benefit analysis before seeking ERP. In addition, a review of the literature may help the patient understand the benefits.

One of the most important elements of combined treatment is communication between the different providers. Both clinicians benefit from information about the complementary treatment. Patients should sign a release of information allowing the collaborating clinicians to exchange information. In the case of OCD there are several important questions to consider, including:

Questions to ask the psychotherapist

- *How willing has the patient been to participate in ERP?*
- *How complicated is the patient's hierarchy?*
- *Where are you at in the hierarchy?*
- *What have you successfully worked through in ERP?*
- *What symptoms have you noticed during ERP?*
- *How are the scores on the Yale-Brown Obsessive Compulsive Scale (Y-BOCS)?*
- *How can I help with response prevention?*

Questions to ask the pharmacotherapist

- *What symptoms are you targeting?*
- *How long will you try this medication?*
- *Are you planning any adjustments?*
- *What symptom changes have you noted?*

CLINICAL RECOMMENDATIONS

On the basis of the issues described earlier, we would recommend the following treatment approach for OCD. In patients with mild to moderate symptoms who are able to function reasonably well, the initial intervention is CBT/ERP. In studies, a decrease of 25% to 30% on the Y-BOCS, a standardized scale to measure OCD symptoms, would reflect response. If this level of response is not achieved after 13 to 20 ERP sessions, combined treatment should be considered.[17] Additionally, if a patient presents with moderate to severe symptoms (including poor insight) or CBT/ERP is not feasible, we would then consider an SSRI. After a trial at maximally tolerated doses for at least 12 weeks, the next pharmacologic trial would be an alternate SSRI.

It is important to open a discussion when you are adjusting or switching to a new medication.

Possible discussion points include:

- *We have tried multiple medications that haven't helped you or you couldn't tolerate.*
- *Your symptoms are still disabling, problematic, unacceptable, or interfere with your ability to accomplish things in your life.*
- *I think at this point we should build on what we have already achieved and get you to a more comfortable level.*

Alternative strategies for those patients where CBT is not accessible include self-help books,[18–22] support groups, and, more recently, the introduction of telephone treatment. In regard to this last option, several studies examined the use of telephone CBT/ERP and found significant reductions in the Y-BOCS scores before and after acute treatment, as well as at 6 months follow-up.[23–25] In addition, those who are less familiar with CBT/ERP can review several books to learn the techniques and how to conduct the sessions.[26,27]

If the patient presents with a comorbid psychiatric disorder (e.g., depression) or has not benefited from one adequate CBT trial or two adequate SSRI trials (i.e., higher doses for at least 12 weeks), then we would combine CBT with an SSRI. With comorbid depression, CBT would focus initially on the depressive symptoms. This is in part based on the observation by Abramowitz et al. that ERP is not as beneficial for depressed patients because these symptoms block the needed decrease in anxiety that results from the exposure.[28]

In more resistant presentations, dual-acting agents such as venlafaxine, mirtazapine, or clomipramine should be considered. Given the more benign adverse effect profile of the first two agents, we would prescribe them before a trial with clomipramine. These dual-acting agents may be used as monotherapy or combined with ERP/CBT or CT.

An alternate strategy would be to combine different medications. The use of an SGA as an augmentation to the primary agent would be a reasonable next step.[29,30] Although other medication combinations have been suggested, the evidence to support such approaches is preliminary. Finally, in the most severely disabled, treatment-resistant patients, (i.e., >5 years duration, multiple failed adequate medication trials, including clomipramine and

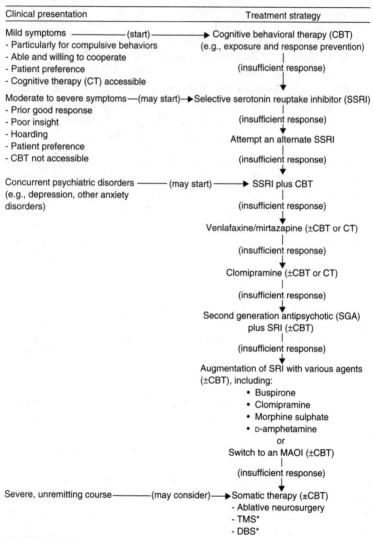

| Clinical presentation | Treatment strategy |

Mild symptoms ————————(start)————————► Cognitive behavioral therapy (CBT)
- Particularly for compulsive behaviors   (e.g., exposure and response prevention)
- Able and willing to cooperate
- Patient preference   (insufficient response)
- Cognitive therapy (CT) accessible

Moderate to severe symptoms—(may start)►Selective serotonin reuptake inhibitor (SSRI)
- Prior good response
- Poor insight   (insufficient response)
- Hoarding   Attempt an alternate SSRI
- Patient preference
- CBT not accessible   (insufficient response)

Concurrent psychiatric disorders ————— (may start) ————► SSRI plus CBT
(e.g., depression, other anxiety
disorders)   (insufficient response)

                                                        Venlafaxine/mirtazapine (±CBT or CT)

                                                                (insufficient response)

                                                         Clomipramine (±CBT or CT)

                                                                (insufficient response)

                                                 Second generation antipsychotic (SGA)
                                                             plus SRI (±CBT)

                                                                (insufficient response)

                                             Augmentation of SRI with various agents
                                             (±CBT), including:
                                                         • Buspirone
                                                         • Clomipramine
                                                         • Morphine sulphate
                                                         • ᴅ-amphetamine
                                                                        or
                                                  Switch to an MAOI (±CBT)

                                                                (insufficient response)

Severe, unremitting course————(may consider)——►Somatic therapy (±CBT)
                                                               - Ablative neurosurgery
                                                               - TMS*
                                                               - DBS*

*Not FDA approved.

FIGURE 3-1 ▦ Treatment strategy for obsessive compulsive disorder. SRI, selective reuptake inhibitor; MAOI, monoamine oxidase inhibitor; TMS, transcranial magnetic stimulation; DBS, deep brain stimulation; FDA, U.S. Food and Drug Administration. (Adapted from Janicak PG, Davis JM, Preskorn SH, et al. *Principles and practice of Psychopharmacotherapy*, 4th ed. Philadelphia: Lippincott Williams & Wilkins; 2006.)[31]

an MAOI; severe disability) treatments such as TMS, DBS, and ablative neurosurgery may be helpful. As with pharmacotherapy, CBT may also complement these procedures.

 Ms. V successfully tolerated exposure that included touching door knobs and sitting on the bus without washing. She no longer avoided public transportation and was traveling by bus at least four times a week. In addition, her showers were reduced to 15 minutes and to once a day. In collaboration with the patient, the family was instructed how to handle her rituals and avoid reassuring her. The patient continued to experience fears of contamination but her functioning improved due to the increased time available for daily activities.

Figure 3-1 outlines the approach we would recommend for treatment of OCD.

Learning points

- ERP is considered the psychotherapeutic treatment of choice for OCD.
- For patients with mild to moderate symptoms who are able to function reasonably well, the initial intervention is CBT/ERP alone.
- For patients with moderate to severe symptoms (including poor insight) or for whom CBT/ERP is not feasible, consider an SSRI alone.
- In more resistant cases, the combination of CBT/ERP plus an SSRI may provide more adequate benefit.

REFERENCES

1. Wheaton M, Cromer K, Lasalle-Ricci VH, et al. Characterizing the hoarding phenotype in individuals with OCD: Associations with cormobidity, severity and gender. *J Anxiety Disord*. 2007;2:12 epub.
2. Samuels JF, Bienvenu OJ III, Pinto A, et al. Hoarding in obsessive-compulsive disorder: results from the OCD collaborative genetics study. *Behav Res Ther*. 2007;45(4):673–686.

3. Lochner C, Kinnear CJ, Hemmings SM, et al. Hoarding in obsessive compulsive disorder: Clinical and genetic correlates. *J Clin Psychiatry.* 2005;66(9):1155–1160.

4. Samuels J, Shugart YY, Grados MA, et al. Significant linkage to compulsive hoarding on chromosome 14 in families with obsessive compulsive disorder: Results from the OCD Collaborative Genetics Study. *Am J Psychiatry.* 2007;164(3):493–499.

5. Saxena S, Brody AL, Maidment KM, et al. Paroxetine treatment of compulsive hoarding. *J Psychiat Res.* 2007;41(6):481–487.

6. Fontenelle LF, Nascimento AL, Mendlowicz MV, et al. An update on the pharmacological treatment of obsessive-compulsive disorder. *Expert Opin Pharmacother.* 2007;8(5):563–583.

7. Janicak PG, Davis JM, Preskorn SH, et al. *Principles and practice of psychopharmacotherapy,* 4th ed. Philadelphia: Lippincott Williams & Wilkins; 2006:1–18.

8. Pigott TA, Seay SM. A review of the efficacy of selective serotonin reuptake inhibitors in obsessive-compulsive disorder. *J Clin Psychiatry.* 1999;60(2):101–106.

9. Koran LM, Hanna GL, Hollander E, et al. Practice guideline for the treatment of patients with obsessive-compulsive disorder. *Am J Psychiatry.* 2007;164(Suppl 7):22.

10. Abramowitz JS. The psychological treatment of obsessive-compulsive disorder. *Can J Psychiatry.* 2006;51:407–416.

11. Sudak D. *Cognitive behavioral therapy for clinicians. Psychotherapy in clinical practice.* Lippincott Williams & Wilkins; 2006.

12. Meyer V. Modification of expectations in cases with obsessional rituals. *Behav Res Ther.* 1966;4:273–280.

13. Abramowitz JS. Effectiveness of psychological and pharmacological treatments for obsessive compulsive disorder: A quantitative review. *J Consult Clin Psychol.* 1997;65:44–52.

14. Cottraux J, Mollard E, Bouvard M, et al. A controlled study of fluvoxamine and exposure in obsessive compulsive disorder. *Int Clin Psychopharmacol.* 1990;5:17–30.

15. O'Connor K, Todorov C, Robillard S, et al. Cognitive-behavior therapy and medication in the treatment of obsessive-compulsive disorder: A controlled study. *Can J Psychiatry.* 1999;44:64–71.

16. O'Connor KP, Aardema F, Robillard S, et al. Cognitive behaviour therapy and medication in the treatment of obsessive-compulsive disorder. *Acta Psychiatr Scand.* 2006;113:408–419.

17. March JS, Frances A, Kahn DA. The expert consensus guideline series: treatment of obsessive compulsive disorder. *J Clin Psychiatry.* 1997;58(Suppl 4):11–28.

18. Steketee G, Pigott TA. *Obsessive compulsive disorder: the latest assessment and treatment strategies.* Dean Psych Press Corporation; 2006.

19. Neziroglu F, Bubrick J, Yaryura-Tobias JA. *Overcoming compulsive hoarding: why you save and how you can stop it*. Oakland: New Harbinger; 2004.

20. Hyman BM, Pedrick C. *The OCD workbook: your guide to breaking free from obsessive compulsive disorder*, 2nd ed. Oakland: New Harbinger; 2005.

21. Grayson J. *Freedom from obsessive-compulsive disorder*. New York: Berkley Books; 2003.

22. Foa EB, Wilson R. *Stop obsessing!: how to overcome your obsessions and compulsions*. Revised ed. New York: Bantam Books; 2001.

23. Lovell K, Fullove L, Garvery R, et al. Telephone treatment of obsessive compulsive disorder. *Behav Cogn Psychother*. 2000;28:87–91.

24. Taylor S, Thordarson DS, Spring T, et al. Telephone administered cognitive behavior therapy for obsessive compulsive disorder. *Cogn Behav Ther*. 2003;32:13–25.

25. Lovell K, Cox D, Haddock G, et al. Telephone administered cognitive behavior therapy for treatment of obsessive compulsive disorder: Randomized controlled noninferiority trial. *Br Med J*. 2006:333(7574):883.

26. Barlow DH. *Clinical handbook of psychological disorders*. New York: The Guilford Press; 2007:209–264.

27. Griest JH. *Obsessive compulsive disorder: a guide*, 5th ed. Madison: Madison Institute of Medicine; 2000.

28. Abramowitz J, Foa E. Does comorbid major depressive disorder influence outcomes of exposure and response prevention for OCD? *Behav Ther*. 2000;31:795–800.

29. Bloch MH, Landeros-Weisenberger A, Kelmendi B, et al. A systematic review: Antipsychotic augmentation with treatment refractory obsessive-compulsive disorder. *Mol Psychiatry*. 2006;11(7): 622–632.

30. Walsh KH, Scott EL, McDougle CJ. The use of antipsychotics in the treatment of obsessive compulsive disorder. *Psychopharmacol Rev*. 2008;43(4):27–34.

31. Janicak PG, Davis JM, Preskorn SH, et al. *Principles and practice of psychopharmacotherapy*, 4th ed. Philadelphia: Lippincott Williams & Wilkins; 2006.

SUGGESTED READINGS

Abramowitz JS, Franklin ME, Schwartz SA, et al. Symptom presentation and outcome of cognitive behavioral therapy for obsessive compulsive disorder. *J Consult Clin Psychol*. 2003;71:1049–1057.

Fisher JR, O'Donohue WT, eds. *Practitioner's guide to evidence-based psychotherapy*. New York, NY: Springer; 2006.

Goodman WK, Price LH, Rasmussen SA. The Yale-Brown obsessive compulsive scale. *Arch Gen Psychiatry*. 1989;46(1):1006–1011.

Greist JH, Bandelow B, Hollander E, et al. WCA recommendations for the long-term treatment of obsessive-compulsive disorder in adults. *CNS Spectr*. 2003;8(Suppl 1):7–16.

March JS, Frances A, Carpenter D. Treatment of obsessive compulsive disorder. Expert consensus panel for obsessive-compulsive disorder. *J Clin Psychiatry*. 1997;58(Suppl 4):2–72.

Panic Disorder

LEARNING OBJECTIVES

The reader will be able to:

1. Understand the differences and relationship between pharmacotherapy and psychotherapy for the treatment of panic disorder (PD).
2. Develop strategies for combined or sequenced treatment approaches for PD.
3. Enhance skills to negotiate these treatment approaches with patients.

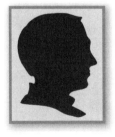

Mr. Y

Mr. Y is a 27-year-old, single man who presented to his primary care physician (PCP) with recent-onset panic attacks. The patient denied a prior psychiatric history. His PCP ruled out any medical causes for his symptoms and prescribed sertraline (starting at 50 mg per day). The patient experienced only a mild reduction in symptoms despite increasing the dose of sertraline to 200 mg per day and continued to experience panic attacks at least twice a week. His PCP then referred him for psychotherapy.

Panic disorder (PD) is a debilitating disease. The estimated lifetime prevalence is 1.5% to 3.5% with an eightfold increased risk in first-degree relatives. The disorder has a bimodal peak in adolescence and mid 30s and may predispose to the development of *other mental disorders* (e.g., other anxiety disorders, mood disorders). Women are twice as likely as men to develop PD. One third to one half of patients will also suffer from *agoraphobia*. Other potential complications are a higher risk of *substance abuse* (perhaps as an attempt to self-medicate), *suicide*, and *mitral valve prolapse*. Because symptoms also overlap with many *physical conditions*, there is often an excessive use of medical services. PD typically follows a waxing and waning course but up to 20% of patients will experience a more chronic, persistent course.

PD consists of several components, including:

- *Panic attack* (at least two episodes that are unexpected, spontaneous)
  - Limited symptoms
  - Full episodes
- *Anticipatory anxiety* for at least 1 month that another episode will occur in certain places or situations
- *Phobic avoidance* of the feared situational trigger(s)
- *Anxiety* about serious medical problems

Table 4-1 lists common symptoms associated with a panic attack.

DIFFERENTIAL DIAGNOSIS

Comorbidity with other psychiatric disorders and overlapping symptoms is common (e.g., 50% to 60% of patients with PD will also meet criteria for major depressive disorder, many patients will experience panic symptoms during a depressive episode). In addition, a variety of other psychiatric and nonpsychiatric disorders may produce panic symptoms, including:

- *Substance-induced* (e.g., caffeine intoxication, alcohol withdrawal)

TABLE 4-1	*ᵃSymptoms of a Panic Attack*

- Shortness of breath/smothering sensations
- Dizziness, unsteady feelings, or faintness
- Palpitations/tachycardia
- Trembling/shaking
- Sweating
- Choking
- Nausea/abdominal distress
- Depersonalization/derealization
- Paresthesias
- Flushes/chills
- Chest pain or discomfort
- Fear of dying
- Fear of going crazy or doing something uncontrolled

ᵃAt least four of these symptoms should be present to meet diagnostic criteria.

- *Medical disorders* (e.g., hyperthyroidism)
- *Other psychiatric disorders* (e.g., major depression, posttraumatic stress disorder, specific phobia, social phobia)

Therefore, a thorough history and physical examination should be conducted to rule out other potential causes.

Mr. Y reported numerous episodes where he suddenly experienced a feeling of pressure in his chest, shortness of breath, sweating, nausea, and fear that he was having a heart attack. Prior to seeing his PCP, he had been to the emergency room on several occasions where he was diagnosed with panic attacks. Although he had anticipatory anxiety he had not begun to avoid situations. Mr. Y denied symptoms of depressed mood or loss of interest. He met criteria for PD without agoraphobia.

NEUROBIOLOGY OF PANIC DISORDER

Environmental and biological factors predispose to the development of this disorder. For example, most symptomatic patients will report a *major life stressor* in the previous year. In addition, PD appears to have the highest level of *family aggregation* (i.e., almost a sevenfold increased risk) among the anxiety disorders. *Twin studies* also indicate that PD has the highest heritability of all the anxiety disorders.

The characteristic *respiratory symptoms* (e.g., dyspnea, rapid breathing) that often accompany panic attacks have led to different hypotheses, including:

- *Respiratory instability* secondary to abnormal brain stem mechanisms
  - Hyperventilation syndrome
  - Increased respiratory variability
  - "False suffocation alarm"
- *Conditioned fear* response
  - Driven by an oversensitive network involving the amygdala, prefrontal cortex, and hypothalamus
  - Physiological changes trigger panic attacks by contributing to the perception of anxiety

In part, on the basis of the putative mechanisms of action of various effective treatments for PD and imaging studies, abnormalities in *neurotransmitter systems* such as *serotonin* and *γ-aminobutyric acid* (*GABA*) have also been implicated.

TREATMENT OF PANIC DISORDER

Pharmacotherapy for Panic Disorder

While benzodiazepines (BZDs) have been used for decades to treat the symptoms of PD, they have largely been replaced by antidepressant agents.[1] As with obsessive compulsive disorder (OCD), the *selective serotonin reuptake inhibitors* (SSRIs) are the recommended first-line drug strategy primarily due to their better safety–tolerability profiles (see Table 2-5 for more details regarding the adverse effects of antidepressants [ADs]). Table 4-2 lists the various classes of drugs frequently used to treat PD. Often, higher doses and longer durations of exposure

TABLE 4-2	*Medications for Treatment of Panic Disorder*	
Class/Generic Name	**Common Trade Name**	**Usual Dose Range (mg/d)**
Benzodiazepines		
Alprazolam	Xanax	2–6
Alprazolam XR	Xanax XR	2–6
Clonazepam	Klonopin	1–2
SSRIs		
Paroxetine	Paxil	40
Paroxetine CR	Paxil CR	40
Fluoxetine	Prozac	20
Sertraline	Zoloft	50
[a]Citalopram	Celexa	20–30
[a]Escitalopram	Lexapro	10
SNRIs		
Venlafaxine ER	Effexor ER	75–225
[a]Duloxetine	Cymbalta	30–120
Tetracyclics		
Mirtazapine	Remeron	7.5–45
Tricyclics		
Imipramine	Tofranil	100–300
Clomipramine	Anafranil	25–150
MAOIs		
[a]Phenelezine	Nardil	15–45
[a]Tranylcypromine	Parnate	15–70

[a]Not approved by U.S. Food and Drug Administration.
SSRIs, selective serotonin reuptake inhibitors; SNRIs, serotonin norepinephrine reuptake inhibitors; MAOIs, monoamine oxidase inhibitors.

(e.g., ≥12 weeks) are required to achieve optimal control of acute symptoms. Additionally, there is growing evidence that these agents are also effective in maintaining symptom control, preventing recurrence, and improving overall functioning in patients with PD.

The BZDs may also be effective monotherapies, but are increasingly used to augment the effects of ADs when response is insufficient or to decrease adverse effects associated with ADs (e.g., agitation, anxiety). Thus, although ADs are usually effective in controlling the panic attacks, BZDs (or psychotherapy) may be necessary to address the anticipatory anxiety and phobic avoidance components of PD. In this context, *alprazolam XR* avoids the more frequent dosing schedule required with its immediate release formulation and may also decrease interdose "breakthrough" anxiety. *Clonazepam* also appears to be a viable alternative BZD (see Chapter 10 for discussion of BZD-related adverse effects).

Antiepileptic drugs (AEDs) and *second-generation antipsychotics* (*SGAs*) (e.g., olanzapine) have also shown promise in preliminary case reports and small trials but await more definitive data before they can be recommended.

Psychotherapy for Panic Disorder

Cognitive behavioral therapy (CBT) is the most empirically validated psychotherapy for PD. Frequently, however, pharmacotherapy is the first treatment approach because patients initially present to their PCP. The CBT strategies that show the most robust effect include combined *cognitive restructuring* and *interoceptive exposure.*[2] The theoretical model for CBT is based on the tenet that a fear of anxiety and the associated physical sensations maintain the disorder. In addition, agoraphobia often develops as the patient begins to avoid situations associated with a panic attack. CBT includes both cognitive and behavioral techniques aimed at understanding and reducing fear of anxiety. This intervention has been successful in both *individual and group formats.* Duration of treatment will vary depending on the presenting symptoms. Although the average number of sessions in treatment studies is 10 to 20, research and clinical experience also support the efficacy of shorter interventions (e.g., six sessions). Because psychosocial stressors such as marital discord are associated with poor response, it is usually necessary to include the family and/or the spouse in treatment.

A typical treatment session includes several phases. The first step is *educating the patients* about their physical symptoms to develop a better understanding of the body's natural response to stress. Once the model is presented, treatment focuses on *exposure to physical symptoms*. In this context, patients monitor symptoms of anxiety and panic attacks to help with treatment planning. Treatment then focuses on *expanding alternative coping skills* (e.g., breathing, retraining, and relaxation) to reduce symptoms. Once a clear picture of the fears and panic are established and patients have developed alternate coping skills, treatment involves exposure to the avoided situations or to the feared physical symptoms. The exposures are designed to test negative thoughts about what is happening to their body and to diminish fearful associations with triggering situations. *Interoceptive exposure* involves repeatedly recreating the feared physical sensations. Techniques may include breathing through a straw, spinning in a chair, running in place and/or hyperventilating. *In vivo exposure* is done in a gradual manner using an avoidance hierarchy. It is important to eliminate any safety behaviors during the exposure (e.g., carrying a bottle of water, having a BZD available). Gradually, the patients place themselves in situations previously avoided without any safety behaviors. *Cognitive restructuring* is another important intervention weaved throughout all these steps. It helps patients realistically view their bodily sensations, understand that their thoughts are only that and identify any unrealistic thoughts.

Combined Psychotherapy and Pharmacotherapy for Panic Disorder

The outcomes of efficacy studies with combined CBT and pharmacotherapy are mixed. For example, Mitte[3] found no significant differences in efficacy between CBT alone and a combination of CBT and pharmacotherapy. Several recent meta-analyses, however, conclude that combining pharmacotherapy with psychotherapy generally produces a better outcome. For example, in a meta-analysis of 21 studies Furukawa et al.[4,5] determined that either combined therapy or CBT alone is an appropriate first-line treatment for PD with or without agoraphobia. Although both approaches appear effective in the short term, some studies found

CBT better for long-term efficacy. In a preliminary trial, Barlow[6] examined sequential treatment options for the treatment of PD and found a trend for CBT nonresponders to further improve with the addition of paroxetine.

Assessing the benefit of combined treatment is slightly more complicated due to the rapid symptom relief associated with medications. The concern is that patients will attribute success to the effects of these medications instead of the addition of coping skills or cognitive techniques or the additive effect from both. This may in part explain why longer-term CBT appears to be more effective.

Given these mixed results, it is crucial for multiple providers to communicate frequently and plan the treatment strategy together.

Questions to ask the psychotherapist

- *What symptoms are you targeting?*
- *Will you be doing any exposure in sessions?*
- *If we plan on making any treatment changes, can we check with each other?*
- *What is your time frame for treatment?*

Questions to ask the pharmacotherapist

- *What symptoms are you targeting?*
- *Are you planning any medication adjustments?*
- *To test the patient's belief that the medication is the only thing working, I may have the patient hold the p.r.n. (as needed) use of the BZD. Do you have any concerns?*
- *What symptom changes have you noted?*
- *How long are you advising the patient to use BZDs?*

Introducing Combined Treatment

Mr. Y had no prior psychiatric history and his current state was very distressing. At the same time, he had difficulty seeing this as a psychological issue and struggled with the belief that he had a medical problem. He experienced some symptom relief with sertraline but the weekly panic attacks continued to interfere with his life (e.g., he was always worried about when the next one would occur). His PCP was able to reassure him that he was in good physical condition and suggested there were other ways to cope with his symptoms. His PCP also discussed working closely with a psychiatrist who had the appropriate expertise and suggested that Mr. Y go for an evaluation. Following a signed release of information, the PCP contacted the psychiatrist and informed him of the patient's concerns. This information facilitated the incorporation of more education about PD during the initial consultation.

Possible discussion points include:

- ■ *I want to reinforce that your physical symptoms are quite real. These symptoms are a very natural response to stress and anxiety.*

- ■ *My concern is that you interpret these symptoms to mean something that is not likely to happen. I want to work with you to learn whether you are misinterpreting these experiences.*

- ■ *I have experience helping people with panic attacks and been successful in reducing them. You have some success with the antidepressant, but I think we can work together so you feel even better.*

- ■ *You and I will work to understand your panic attacks and find ways to lessen their severity, hopefully stopping them completely.*

- ■ *We will continue to check on your medication and may adjust the dose, but we are also going to work on other ways to cope with your symptoms.*

For patients who do not have available resources there are alternative options to CBT and several self-help workbooks. For example, studies have reported improvement with *telephone, videoconference-guided exposure and skill training,* or *Internet treatment.*[7,8] It is important to note that research has found that the self-help interventions were the most successful with highly motivated patients but those with more severe symptoms required therapist contact. Graham[9] recommends selecting self-help books with proven efficacy and usefulness to the reader. *Mastery of Your Anxiety and Panic* by Barlow and Craske[10] is directed at patients but also has an accompanying book for therapists. As part of their *Overcoming Series,* Silove and Manicavasagar[11] provide a self-help guide using CBT for PD. There are also books available for coping with general anxiety, including *10 Simple Solutions to Worry* by Gyoerkoe and Wiegartz.[12] For those unfamiliar with CBT, Barlow outlines its history, assessment, and treatment of PD.[6]

Mr. Y continued combined treatment for 4 months. By developing a better understanding of stress, increasing relaxation skills with progressive muscle relaxation, challenging beliefs about his physical symptoms, and exposure to the physical symptoms of an increased heart rate, he no longer experienced panic attacks. On occasion, however, he focused on a strange sensation associated with his heart beat. The hypervigilance was successfully targeted during several booster sessions. After 2 more asymptomatic months, he discontinued the sertraline.

CLINICAL RECOMMENDATIONS

We recommend the following treatment approach for PD. In mild attacks (e.g., low frequency, less severe symptoms), we would start with CBT which includes education, gradual exposure to the feared object or situation, training in relaxation techniques, and cognitive restructuring. In these situations, CBT has been very successful with up to 75% of patients becoming panic-free following treatment. If insufficient or the symptoms are moderate in intensity, we would consider a trial with an SSRI alone or combined with CBT if medication also proves to be insufficient. With more severe symptoms, we would introduce a BZD in combination with CBT and, if necessary, add an SSRI to manage more persistent symptoms. In resistant cases, we would consider switching from an SSRI to a tricyclic antidepressant (TCA) or monoamine oxidase inhibitor (MAOI) in addition to CBT (with or without a BZD). Other approaches may include the use of certain AEDs (e.g., gabapentin, valproate). In these strategies, it is important to open a discussion when you are introducing combined treatment, adjusting doses, or switching to a new medication.

Possible discussion points include:

- *We have tried several medications that were helpful but you continue to experience symptoms or side effects.*
- *You have been very successful in developing new skills. You understand your symptoms of stress and you scan your body much less frequently. In addition, your general tension is reduced significantly.*
- *Let us compare your anxiety scores when you started and your present scores. You have made great progress. I am wondering if there are other things we can do to help with your symptoms. This might be a time to discuss adding medication.*

■ *At this point we should build on what we have achieved and increase your comfort level.*

Figure 4-1 outlines the approach we are recommending for PD.

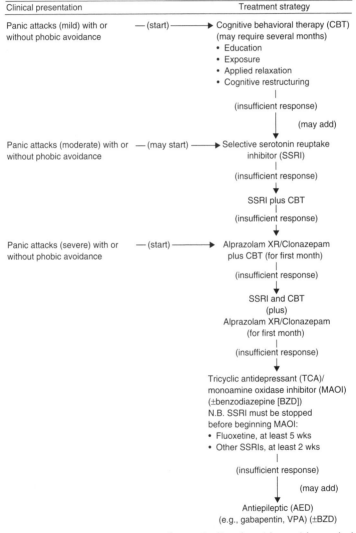

FIGURE 4-1 ■ Treatment strategy for panic disorder with or without phobic avoidance. VPA, valproic acid. (Adapted from Janicak PG, Davis JM, Preskorn SH, et al. *Principles and Practice of Psychopharmacotherapy*, 4th ed. Philadelphia: Lippincott Williams & Wilkins; 2006:529.)[13]

Learning points

- CBT or an SSRI may be appropriate first-line treatment for mild to moderately severe PD.
- More severe symptoms of PD usually require medication initially, including an SSRI with or without a BZD.
- Persistent symptoms may benefit from combined pharmacotherapy and psychotherapy.

REFERENCES

1. Katon WJ. Panic disorder. *N Engl J Med*. 2006;354:22.
2. Gould RA, Otto M, Pollack MH. A meta-analysis of treatment outcome for panic disorder. *Clin Psychol Rev*. 1995;15(8):819–844.
3. Mitte K. A meta-analysis of the efficacy of psycho- and pharmacotherapy in panic disorder with and without agoraphobia. *J Affect Disord*. 2005;88:27–45.
4. Furukawa TA, Watanabe N, Churchill R. Psychotherapy plus antidepressant for panic disorder with or without agoraphobia: A systematic review. *Br J Psychiatry*. 2006;188:305–312.
5. Furukawa TA, Watanabe N, Churchill R. Psychotherapy plus antidepressants for panic disorder with or without agoraphobia. *Cochrane Database Syst Rev*. 2007;24(1):CD004364.
6. Barlow DH. *Clinical handbook of psychological disorders*. New York: The Guilford Press; 2007:1–64.
7. Bouchard S, Paquin B, Payeur R, et al. Delivering cognitive behavior therapy for panic disorder with agoraphobia in videoconference. *Telemed J E Health*. 2004;10(1):13–24.
8. Carlbring P, Ekselius L, Andersson G. Treatment of panic disorder via the Internet: A randomized trial of CBT vs relaxation. *J Behav Ther Exp Psychiatry*. 2003;34:129–140.
9. Graham Reading about self-help books on obsessive compulsive and anxiety disorders—a review. *psychiatric bull*. 2003;27:235–237.
10. Barlow DH, Craske MG. *Mastery of your anxiety and panic*. New York: Oxford Press; 2007.
11. Silove D, Manicavasagar V. *Overcoming Panic: a self-help guide using cognitive behavioral techniques*. New York: New York University Press; 2001.
12. Gyoerkoe KL, Wiegartz PS. *10 simple solutions to worry: how to calm your mind, relax your body and reclaim your life*. Oakland: New Harbinger; 2006.

13. Janicak PG, Davis JM, Preskorn SH, et al. *Principles and practice of psychopharmacotherapy*, 4th ed. Philadelphia: Lippincott Williams & Wilkins; 2006.

SUGGESTED READINGS

American Psychiatric Association. Practice guideline for the treatment of patients with panic disorder. Work group on panic disorder. *Am J Psychiatry.* 1998;155(Suppl 5):1–34.

Bandelow B, Seidler-Brander U, Becker A, et al. Meta-analysis of randomized controlled comparisons of psychopharmacological and psychological treatments for anxiety disorders. *World J Biol Psychiatry.* 2007;8(3):175–187.

Barlow DH, Gorman JM, Shear MK, et al. Cognitive-behavioral therapy, imipramine, or their combination for *panic* disorder: A randomized controlled trial. *JAMA.* 2000;283(19)2529–2536.

Barlow DH, Craske MG. *Mastery of your anxiety and panic: Therapist Guide.* New York: Oxford Press; 2007.

Burns DD. *When Panic Attacks: the new drug free anxiety therapy that can change your life.* Broadway books: New york; 2007.

Campbell-Sills L, Stein MB. *Guideline watch: practice guideline for the treatment of patients with panic disorder.* Arlington: American Psychological Association; 2006.

Fisher JR, O'Donohue WT, eds. *Practitioner's guide to evidence-based psychotherapy.* New York, NY: Springer; 2006.

Graham Reading about self-help books on obsessive compulsive and anxiety disorders – a review. *Psychopharmacol Bull.* 2003;27:235–237.

Gyoerkoe KL, Wiegartz PS. *10 simple solutions to worry: how to calm your mind, relax your body and reclaim your life.* New Harbinger: Oakland; 2006.

Wantanabe N, Churchill R, Furukawa TA. Combination of psychotherapy and benzodiazepines versus either therapy alone for panic disorder: A systematic review. *BMC Psychiatry.* 2007;7:18.

Posttraumatic Stress Disorder

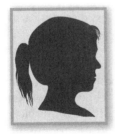

Ms. U

Ms. U is a 22-year-old, single woman who presented with symptoms of depression following a sexual assault during her senior year in college. She began to experience periods of sadness and crying, loss of sleep, loss of energy, and feelings that she did not want to live. Ms. U also reported flashbacks, a sense of hypervigilance and feeling "on edge." Ms. U had no prior psychiatric history. She was experiencing difficulty finding a job and pursuing her career following graduation.

Posttraumatic stress disorder (PTSD) involves reexperiencing a severe trauma with intense fear, helplessness, or horror accompanied by increased arousal and avoidance of any associated stimuli. These symptoms should persist for at least 1 month and cause significant disability. Events that may precipitate this condition include:

- *Combat*
- Violent personal *assault* (e.g., rape)
- *Kidnapping*
- *Torture*
- *Hostage* taking
- Natural or man-made *disasters* (e.g., Hurricane Katrina, September 11, 2001)
- Severe *accidents* (*e.g., brain trauma secondary to an explosion*)
- Life-threatening *illness*

Symptoms of PTSD may include:

- *Reexperiencing* (memories or "flashbacks" of the event)
- *Avoidance*/numbing
  - Avoiding stimuli that bring back memories
  - Feeling numb or emotionless
  - Withdrawal from social contact
  - Abuse of alcohol or other drugs
- *Hyperarousal*
  - Easily startled
  - Angry outbursts
  - Feeling "on guard" or irritable

Although 50% or more of the population may experience a traumatic event, most do not develop acute stress disorder (ASD) or PTSD. The National Comorbidity Survey (NCS) estimates the lifetime prevalence of PTSD at 7.8%. The female to male lifetime prevalence ratio is 2:1. This syndrome is also associated with significant disability (e.g., occupational, psychosocial) and occurs more frequently in those with prior adverse childhood experiences or acomorbid diagnosis. There is also a high comorbidity with other psychiatric disorders (e.g., major depression, substance abuse). In addition, there is an increased suicide risk.

Recently, the criteria for PTSD have been questioned with data finding equal percentages of patients with or without a history of trauma meeting the other inclusion criteria based on the Diagnostic and Statistical Manual of Mental Disorders-IV (DSM-IV).[1] Malingering has also been raised as a possible basis for this diagnosis in up to 50% of cases.[2] These observations have led to discussions about making the criteria for PTSD more restrictive to improve their reliability.

DIFFERENTIAL DIAGNOSIS

With PTSD, the event must be extreme. By contrast, *adjustment disorder* can involve a stressor at any level of severity. *ASD* must occur within 4 weeks of the event, last at least 2 days, involve dissociative symptoms during or immediately after the event, and resolve during that 4-week time frame. *Obsessive compulsive disorder (OCD)* and *malingering* are also differential diagnostic considerations. Symptoms of PTSD can also overlap with concurrent psychiatric problems such as major depressive disorder, other anxiety disorders, and substance use disorders.

Ms. U began to experience significant fear soon after the assault, and stated that she constantly felt like she was in danger or at risk. Because the attack happened near the end of the year, she was able to complete her remaining coursework; however, her concentration was greatly diminished with flashbacks and she began to withdraw to feel safe. After graduating and returning home, she began to experience periods of sadness and crying, diminished energy, weight loss, and feeling hopelessness and helplessness. She began to contemplate suicide, feeling that she would never be the same again. She was terrorized at night with vivid dreams and flashbacks. Ms. U met criteria for both PTSD and a major depressive episode.

NEUROBIOLOGY OF POSTTRAUMATIC STRESS DISORDER

There are potential factors that may predict who will develop ASD or PTSD. They include biological (e.g., genetic, gender), prior traumatic experiences, and specific acute reactions to an event (e.g., dissociation; panic attacks).

Biological predisposition has been explored in the context of genes that regulate:

- The *serotonin* transporter
- *Corticotropin-releasing factor* (CRF)
- Brain-derived *neurotrophic factor* (BDNF)

Imaging studies have identified possible abnormalities in hippocampal volumes associated with increases in regional cerebral blood flow (rCBF) to this area.[3] Further, functional magnetic resonance imaging (fMRI) studies find evidence for an exaggerated amygdalar activity in conjunction with a decreased medial cortical response.[4]

TREATMENT OF POSTTRAUMATIC STRESS DISORDER

Strategies to manage PTSD include both psychotherapy and pharmacotherapy, frequently in combination.

Pharmacotherapy for Posttraumatic Stress Disorder

Antidepressants (*ADs*) represent the pharmacotherapy of choice for PTSD. Because of a substantial controlled trial database and safety–tolerability profile, selective serotonin reuptake inhibitors (SSRIs) are the preferred class of ADs. Studies indicate that these agents can benefit all three major symptoms (i.e., reexperiencing, avoidance, hyperarousal). Further, they often improve symptoms of comorbid disorders (e.g., depression). More recent short-term and continuation trials with venlafaxine XR have also shown promise. Table 2-4 lists the common adverse effects associated with various ADs.

Benzodiazepines (*BZDs*) are usually add-on agents to help reduce anxiety and improve sleep. Caution in their use, however, is required given the high rates of substance abuse in this population. Chapter 10 discusses other adverse effects of BZDs in more detail.

Second-generation antipsychotics (*SGAs*), certain *antiepileptic drugs* (AEDs) (e.g., lamotrigine, topiramate, divalproex sodium), α_2-*adrenergic agonists* (e.g., clonidine), and *ß-adrenergic antagonists* (e.g., propranolol) have also been studied for the treatment of PTSD. For each of these classes of drugs, the data is more limited and at times contradictory.

Factors that increase risk may help predict who will ultimately develop ASD or PTSD in reaction to severe trauma and allow "preemptive" interruption of the processes of fear conditioning and reconsolidation. Drug candidates for such an approach, include:

- β-Blockers (e.g., propranolol)
- AEDs (e.g., pregabalin)
- CRF-1 antagonists

The idea is to avoid the development of the full syndrome. Preliminary evidence indicates that early recognition and treatment with pharmacotherapy and/or psychotherapy in individuals who have experienced severe trauma and have multiple risk factors for developing ASD or PTSD may be beneficial.

> Ms. U presented with both depressive and PTSD symptoms. Following the initial evaluation we began treatment with paroxetine (20 mg per day) given its approval for treatment of depression and PTSD. The initial focus was to control the depressive symptoms (e.g., suicidal ideation associated with feeling hopeless) with referral for prolonged exposure to more effectively target the specific PTSD symptoms.

Psychotherapy for Posttraumatic Stress Disorder

Several professional societies and guidelines suggest that the first-line treatments for PTSD include prolonged exposure, cognitive processing therapy, stress inoculation training, cognitive therapy, and eye movement desensitization and reprocessing (International Society for Traumatic Stress Studies, US Department of Veterans Affairs, Department of Defense, and American Psychiatric Association). All of these approaches have been empirically tested and involve cognitive processing in one form or another. The empirical support for eye movement desensitization and reprocessing, however, is heavily criticized. Presently, the evidence points to prolonged exposure as the most effective component of these psychotherapies.

In *prolonged exposure therapy* the clinician and patient gradually review the traumatic event in the safe environment of the therapy session so the patient can process the experience including related thoughts and feelings. Sessions typically last longer than a standard encounter to give adequate time to relive the experience, which is key to the success of this intervention.

Cognitive processing therapy, first developed with rape victims, has expanded to include other types of trauma. This cognitive therapy follows a 12-session structured approach conducted in an individual or group format. It involves writing down the traumatic event and then repeatedly reviewing it and the associated thoughts and feelings.

Stress inoculation training is a multiphase intervention also conducted in an individual or group format and includes education about the model and coping skills training. Patients are educated about the body's response to stress and trained in the use of relaxation, thought stopping and cognitive restructuring for example.

Cognitive therapy comes in two forms for PTSD treatment. One focuses on monitoring current symptoms with daily diaries to help the patient develop skills to identify maladaptive thoughts. The second focuses on the thoughts and feelings surrounding the traumatic event and exploring how that event changed the patient's worldview. For example, a patient may feel he or she will never be safe again. The focus of treatment is to examine the distortions associated with this changed perspective.

Eye movement desensitization and reprocessing theory has received much negative attention. It includes eight phases with both cognitive exposure to the trauma and the added component of lateral eye movements. The model proposes that these movements help process the trauma. Although frequently used, this approach has limited empirical support and the data are mixed on its therapeutic components. In addition, other studies report that the eye movement component of this approach is not effective.[5]

Although PTSD is not diagnosed until 1 month following a traumatic event, several studies have found that introducing cognitive behavior therapy (CBT) within the first month of a trauma (e.g., ASD) may reduce symptoms and possibly preclude the full development of PTSD.[6] The research on early intervention, however, has been limited to victims of assault or accidents and needs further validation.

With the increase in the incidence of PTSD in the military and the stigma attached to mental health treatment, *Internet treatment* for PTSD was developed as an option. Litz et al.[7] studied a therapist-driven, online training with CBT in military personnel following the September 11, 2001 attack. At 6-month follow-up, the group treated with CBT had significantly less symptoms of PTSD, depression, and anxiety than the group treated with supportive counseling. Knaevelsrud and Maercker[8] used Internet-based PTSD therapy (based on CBT principles) in a German speaking population and found similar results, concluding that a successful therapeutic relationship can be established with this approach.

 Ms. U was on an AD and continued to experience significant symptoms of PTSD; therefore we focused on symptoms related to the trauma. As suicidal ideation diminished, she was motivated to begin psychotherapy. With multiple issues, the interventions may be more complicated in an effort to balance the patient's needs. Following a thorough introduction of the treatment model, we began prolonged exposure therapy and cognitive processing. During the reliving of the trauma, we worked to recall the events as vividly as possible. The sessions were audiotaped and Ms. U was given homework assignments to listen to the tape between sessions. During the trauma review, maladaptive thoughts or assumptions were targeted and addressed when appropriate. For example, Ms. U felt she should have fought back and blamed herself for not being stronger.

Combined Psychotherapy and Pharmacotherapy for Posttraumatic Stress Disorder

The use of combined treatment for PTSD is complicated. The American Psychiatric Association guidelines suggest the use of ADs (particularly SSRIs) as the initial approach. In this context, there are limited controlled trials and only two medications are presently approved by the U.S. Food and Drug Administration (FDA) for its treatment (i.e., sertraline and paroxetine). Britain's National Institute for Clinical Excellence (NICE) (http://guidance.nice.org.uk), however, supports the use of cognitive therapies as first-line treatment. Depending on availability and patient preference, we believe either approach is supported by the empirical trial data and clinical experience. Combining medication(s) with *prolonged exposure therapy, cognitive processing therapy, stress inoculation training, or cognitive therapy,* however, may produce a more robust and lasting benefit.

Introducing Combined Treatment

 Ms. U was presented with the latest information on the treatment of PTSD and comorbid depression. Following a discussion of treatment options and a risk–benefit analysis, it was decided to continue other AD and refer her to a psychotherapist for prolonged exposure.

Possible discussion points include:

- *It seems that your trauma affects your mood and you are experiencing significant symptoms of depression.*
- *I think that both those issues need to be addressed and we will likely to do that with one medication.*
- *Let me discuss the risks and benefits of medication.*
- *Although the medication may help with both sets of symptoms, there is an additional therapy that can help you cope more effectively with the trauma you experienced.*
- *You can choose either or both of these approaches to help you feel better.*
- *Let us talk about the risks and benefits of the different approaches.*

The coordination of care is very important for successful treatment of complicated cases. If more than one clinician is providing care, it is important for them to remain in contact during treatment. Following a signed release of information, there are several questions that may be useful including:

Questions to ask the psychotherapist
- *What symptoms are you targeting?*
- *What cognitive distortions have you been working with?*
- *As you work through the trauma, what beliefs have changed?*

Questions to ask the pharmacotherapist
- *What medications are you recommending?*
- *What symptoms are you targeting?*
- *What is your recommendation for the use of other agents such as BZDs?*

CLINICAL RECOMMENDATIONS

Our recommendation is to begin with psychotherapy, including *prolonged exposure therapy, cognitive processing therapy, stress inoculation training, or cognitive therapy.* Owing to the high incidence of comorbid anxiety and depression, we suggest a careful diagnostic assessment and symptom-anchored use of medications (e.g., ADs). To control more disabling acute symptoms such as panic and dysomnia, short-term adjunctive BZDs are also reasonable.

Combining medication(s) with *prolonged exposure therapy, cognitive processing therapy, stress inoculation training, or cognitive therapy* may produce a more robust and lasting benefit.

In those patients who continue to experience symptoms, various agents may be beneficial (e.g., clonidine for persistent hyperarousal).

For patients who do not have access to these psychotherapies, there are mixed reports on the use of self-help books. For example, Ehlers et al.[9] reported that self-help treatments may be no more effective than no treatment. In this context there are some guides that may be useful. Foa et al.[10] in the *Treatments That Work Series* recently published prolonged exposure treatment manuals for both therapists and patients. William and Poijula published *The PTSD Workbook.*[11] For those clinicians unfamiliar with the treatment techniques, there are several useful textbooks including the book titled *Effective Treatments for PTSD* by Foa, Keane, and Friedman[12] or Barlow's *Clinical Handbook of Psychological Disorders.*[13] A recent publication by Marks et al.[14] reviews the use of computer-aided psychotherapies for several disorders and is also a useful reference.

 Ms. U's symptoms of depression began to remit with the combination of treatments and prolonged exposure was successful in reducing her trauma-related symptoms. She was no longer experiencing flashbacks and began applying for jobs as her concentration and energy increased. She successfully obtained employment and continued her treatment with paroxetine.

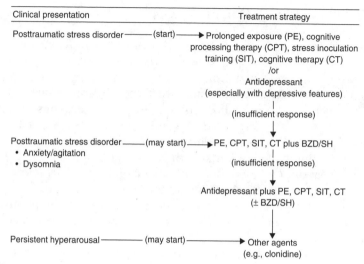

FIGURE 5-1 ■ Treatment strategy for posttraumatic stress disorder. BZD, benzodiazepine, SH, sedative hypnotic. (Adapted from Janicak PG, Davis JM, Preskorn SH, et al. *Principles and Practice of Psychopharmacotherapy*, 4th ed. Philadelphia: Lippincott Williams & Wilkins; 2006:541.)

Figure 5-1 outlines the treatment approach we recommend for PTSD.[15]

Learning points

- Guidelines differ as to whether CBT or pharmacotherapy should be the first-line treatment approach for PTSD.
- Prolonged exposure therapy, cognitive processing therapy, stress inoculation training, or cognitive therapy are the best-studied psychotherapies for PTSD.
- SSRIs and venlafaxine XR are the best-studied pharmacotherapies for PTSD.
- BZDs are useful as adjuncts to manage associated anxiety and dysomnia.
- One of the most effective elements of the psychotherapies appears to be prolonged exposure.
- Combining or sequencing various psychotherapeutic approaches with or without medication may enhance outcomes.

REFERENCES

1. Bodkin JA, Pope HG, Detke MJ, et al. Is PTSD caused by traumatic stress? *J Anxiety Disord*. 2007;21(2):176–182.
2. Rosen GM, Taylor S. Pseudo-PTSD. *J Anxiety Disord*. 2007;21(2): 201–210.
3. Shin LM, Shin PS, Heckers S, et al. Hippocampal function in post-traumatic stress disorder. *Hippocampus*. 2004;14(3):292–300.
4. Shin LM, Wright CI, Cannistraro PA, et al. A functional magnetic resonance imaging study of amygdala and medial prefrontal cortex responses to overtly presented fearful faces in posttraumatic stress disorder. *Arch Gen Psychiatry*. 2005;62(3):273–381.
5. Davidson PR, Parker KH. Eye movement desensitization and reprocessing (EMDR): A meta-analysis. *J Consult Clin Psychol*. 2001; 69(2):305–316.
6. Bryant RA, Moulds ML, Nixon RVD. Cognitive behavior therapy of acute stress disorder: A four year follow-up. *Behav Res Ther*. 2003;41: 489–494.
7. Litz BT, Engel CC, Bryan RA, et. al. A randomized controlled proof-of-concept trial of an internet based, therapist assisted self management treatment for post traumatic stress disorder. *Am J Psychiatry*. 2007;164(11):1676–1683.
8. Knaevelsrud C, Maercker A. Internet-based treatment for PTSD reduces distress and facilitates the development of a strong therapeutic alliance: A randomized controlled clinical trial. *BMC Psychiatry*. 2007;19(7):13.
9. Ehlers A, Clark DM, Hackmann A, et al. A randomized controlled trial of cognitive therapy, a self help booklet, and repeated assessments as early interventions for posttraumatic stress disorder. *Arch Gen Psychiatry*. 2003;60(10):1024–1032.
10. Foa E, Hembree E, Rothbaum B. *Prolonged exposure therapy for PTSD: emotional processing of traumatic experiences therapist guide (treatments that work)*. New York: Oxford University Press; 2007.
11. Williams MB, Poijula S. *The PTSD workbook: simple, effective techniques for overcoming traumatic stress symptoms*. Oakland: New Harbinger Publications; 2002.
12. Foa EB, Keane TM, Friedman MJ. *Effective treatments for PTSD: practice guidelines from the international society for traumatic stress studies*. New York: Guilford Press; 2000.
13. Barlow DH. *Clinical handbook of psychological disorders*. New York: Guilford Press; 2007.
14. Marks IM, Cavanagh K, Gega L. *Hand-on help: computer-aided psychotherapy*. New York Psychology Press; 2007.
15. Janicak PG, Davis JM, Preskorn SH, et al. *Principles and practice of psychopharmacotherapy*, 4th ed. Philadelphia: Lippincott Williams & Wilkins; 2006.

78   INTEGRATING PSYCHOLOGICAL AND BIOLOGICAL THERAPIES

SUGGESTED READINGS

American Psychiatric Association. *Diagnostic and statistical manual of mental disorders DSM-IV-TR*, 4th ed. Washington, DC: American Psychiatric Publishing, Inc.; 2000.

Charney DS. Psychobiological mechanisms of resilience and vulnerability: Implications for successful adaptation to extreme stress. *Am J Psychiatry*. 2004;161(2):195–216.

Davidson J, Baldwin D, Stein DJ, et al. Treatment of posttraumatic stress disorder with venlafaxine extended release: A 6-month randomized controlled trial. *Arch Gen Psychiatry*. 2006;63(10):1158–1165.

Davidson J, Rothbaum BO, Tucker P, et al. Venlafaxine extended release in posttraumatic stress disorder: A sertraline- and placebo-controlled study. *J Clin Psychopharmacol*. 2006;26(3):259–267.

Davis LL, Davidson JR, Ward LC, et al. Divalproex in the treatment of posttraumatic stress disorder: A randomized, double-blind, placebo-controlled trial in a veteran population. *J Clin Psychopharmacol*. 2008;28(1):84–88.

Fisher JR, O'Donohue WT, eds. *Practitioner's guide to evidence-based psychotherapy*. New York, NY: Springer; 2006.

Hairiri AR, Tessitore A, Mattay VS, et al. Serotonin transporter genetic variation and the response of the human amygdala. *Science*. 2002;297(5580):400–403.

Heim C, Newport DJ, Heit S, et al. Pituitary-adrenal and autonomic responses to stress in women after sexual and physical abuse in childhood. *JAMA*. 2000;284(5):592–597.

Mula M, Pini S, Cassano GB. The role of anticonvulsant drugs in anxiety disorders: A critical review of the evidence. *J Clin Psychopharmacol*. 2007;27(3):263–272.

Pitman RK, Sanders KM, Zusman RM, et al. Pilot study of secondary prevention of posttraumatic stress disorder with propranolol. *Biol Psychiatry*. 2002;51(2):189–192.

Rosen GM, Spitzer RL, McHugh PR. Problems with the posttraumatic stress disorder diagnosis and its future in DSM V. *Br J Psychiatry*. 2008;192:3–4.

Schnurr PP, Friedman MJ, Engel CC, et al. Cognitive behavioral therapy for posttraumatic stress disorder in women: a randomized controlled trial. *JAMA*. 2007;297(8):820–830.

Tucker P, Trautmann RP, Wyatt DB, et al. Efficacy and safety of topiramate monotherapy in civilian posttraumatic stress disorder: A randomized, double-blind, placebo-controlled study. *J Clin Psychiatry*. 2007;68(2):201–206.

Tucker P, Zaninelli R, Yehuda R, et al. Paroxetine in the treatment of chronic posttraumatic stress disorder: Results of a placebo-controlled, flexible-dosage trial. *J Clin Psychiatry.* 2001;62(11): 860–868.

Ursano RJ, Bell C, Eth S, et al. Work Group on ASD and PTSD, Steering Committee on Practice Guidelines. Practice guideline for the treatment of patients with acute stress disorder and posttraumatic stress disorder. *Am J Psychiatry.* 2004;161(Suppl 11):3–31.

6

Sleep Disorders

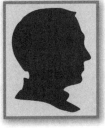

Mr. Z

Mr. Z is a 47-year-old, married man who presented with complaints of insomnia. He has a history of sleep difficulties often associated with life stressors. The typical pattern of his insomnia is to persist for weeks to months before resolution. He has tried several over-the-counter (OTC) sleep aids without success. His primary care physician (PCP) diagnosed him with persistent primary insomnia and prescribed zolpidem (10 mg q.h.s.). Mr. Z had no prior history of psychiatric disorders, obstructive sleep apnea (OSA), seizure disorder, or parasomnias. Because of an incomplete

TABLE 6-1	*Sleep Disorders*

Dysomnias (Primary disorders of initiating or maintaining sleep or excessive sleepiness characterized by problems in the amount, quality, or timing of sleep)

- *Insomnia* (Difficulty initiating or maintaining sleep or not feeling rested after an apparent adequate amount of sleep; ≥1 mo)
  - Primary
  - Secondary
- *Hypersomnia* (Falling asleep easily and unintentionally)
  - Primary
  - Secondary
- *Narcolepsy* (Reported irresistible attacks of sleep, cataplexy, and recurrent intrusions of rapid eye movement [REM] sleep into the transition period between sleep and wakefulness)
- *Breathing-related* (Sleep disruption due to abnormal ventilation during sleep)
  - *Sleep apnea*
- *Circadian rhythm* (Mismatch between normal rest–activity schedule and circadian sleep–wake pattern)

Parasomnias (Abnormal events during sleep, specific sleep stages, or the threshold between sleep and wakefulness)

- *Nightmares* (Repeated occurrence of frightening dreams that cause awakening)
- *Sleep terror* (Abrupt awakenings usually associated with a panicky scream or cry)
- *Sleepwalking* (Repeated episodes of complex motor behavior initiated during sleep)

(Adapted from American Psychiatric Association. *Diagnostic and statistical manual of mental disorders*, 4th ed. Text Revision. Washington, DC: American Psychiatric Association; copyright 2000.)

resolution, he was referred for cognitive behavioral therapy (CBT).

Sleep disorders are prevalent; can be primary or secondary to other psychiatric, psychosocial, substance use, or medical problems; may cause significant physical or psychological symptoms; often go unrecognized; and when diagnosed, may not be adequately managed. The International Classification of Sleep Disorders identifies 88 types, of which insomnia is the most prominent. For example, insomnia is estimated to affect 30% to 40% of the adult population, with more rigorously defined disorders affecting 10% to 15% of the population. Table 6-1 lists the major categories of sleep disorders and provides a brief description of each.

DIFFERENTIAL DIAGNOSIS

There are numerous conditions that may be considered in the differential diagnosis of the various sleep disorders. Disrupted *sleep secondary to a mental disorder, general medical condition, or substance use* are common differential diagnostic considerations for all these disorders.

For *primary insomnia* other considerations may include short sleepers (a normal variant), circadian rhythm sleep disorder, narcolepsy, breathing-related sleep disorder, and parasomnias. For *primary hypersomnia* other considerations are long sleepers (a normal variant), inadequate amount of nocturnal sleep, and primary insomnia. For *narcolepsy*, both sleep deprivation and primary hypersomnia may also cause daytime sleepiness. For *breathing-related* disorders (e.g., OSA) differential considerations are narcolepsy, snoring, and nocturnal panic attacks. For *circadian rhythm* disorder differential considerations are normal patterns of sleep, normal adjustments following a change in schedule, and volitional patterns of delayed sleep hours.

For *nightmare* disorder, the differential diagnoses should include sleep terror, panic attacks, and breathing-related disorders. For *sleep terror* other considerations are nightmares, sleepwalking, seizures, and hypnagogic hallucinations. Finally, for *sleepwalking* disorder other considerations are sleep terror, breathing-related disorder, and sleep-related epilepsy.

Mr. Z and his wife described increasing difficulty falling asleep, tossing and turning during the night, and extreme fatigue during the day. He also reported that his concentration was poor and if things were quiet for a moment he would find himself falling asleep. His PCP ruled out narcolepsy because the episodes were not irresistible periods of sleep onset and there were no episodes of muscle weakness (i.e., cataplexy).

NEUROBIOLOGY OF SLEEP DISORDERS

Because the putative causes for sleep disorders vary depending on the specific type, we briefly describe the major conditions and our understanding of their biological basis.

Insomnia

Although the cause of primary insomnia is poorly understood, one possible factor is an *overengaged arousal system*. Therefore, these patients are more likely to have increased body temperature, elevated metabolic and heart rates, and increased levels of catecholamines. Further, *family aggregation* is a risk factor and suggests a genetic basis. Agents working through the *γ-aminobutyric acid (GABA)$_A$-chloride ion complex* can improve insomnia. For example, *benzodiazepines* (BZDs) bind to the GABA$_A$ receptor α_1 subunit to promote sedation.

More recently, *non-BDZ agents* have become available. They are more selective for the GABA$_A$ α subunit, do not produce active metabolites, and have shorter half-lives compared to the BZDs.

An alternate approach is represented by *ramelteon*, a melatonin receptor type 1 and type 2 agonist. Its action is thought to facilitate the impact of melatonin on circadian rhythms mediated through the suprachiasmatic nucleus of the hypothalamus.

Hypersomnia

Narcolepsy. This is the best known primary disorder of excessive daytime sleepiness (EDS). Although its cause is also not completely understood, various factors may increase the risk of its occurrence including:

- *Immune system* dysfunction
- *Trauma*
- *Hormonal* changes
- *Stress*
- *Gender* (men more than women)
- *Obesity*
- *Familial history* of narcolepsy

The underlying cause appears to be a malfunction in the normal interaction between *sleep and arousal centers* in the central nervous system (CNS). Further, critical to this process is an impairment in the normal activity of the neurotransmitter, *hypocretin*, which is produced by cells in the posterior half of the lateral hypothalamus. The evidence to date indicates that damage to this system, perhaps mediated by an autoimmune process, is the major contributor to narcoleptic symptoms.

Sleep-Related Breathing Disorders. There are three forms of sleep-related breathing disorders (SRBDs), including:

- Blockage of the *oropharynx* (OSA)
- Impair *diaphragmatic* effort (central sleep apnea)
- Secondary to excessive *weight* (central alveolar hypoventilation)

Sleep electroencephalograms (EEGs) often reveal absent or decreased slow-wave sleep or early-onset rapid eye movement (REM) sleep. Long-term adverse effects can include hypertension and vascular events (e.g., myocardial infarction, stroke).

Parasomnias

These disorders are characterized by abnormal events occurring in stage 4 sleep or during transitional periods between sleep and wakefulness.

TREATMENT OF SLEEP DISORDERS

Because most sleep complaints involve the dysomnias and most clinical trials address these specific sleep disorders, we will focus on their treatment.

Pharmacotherapy of Sleep Disorders

Insomnia. *Insomnia* is the most common sleep disorder and we will focus on its treatment with more limited discussion of other dysomnias (e.g., narcolepsy, OSA). Medication approaches are dictated by our understanding of the basis for insomnia that can be divided into three groups: *primary* which represents a small proportion of patients, insomnia as a *symptom* of other specific sleep disorders (e.g., restless leg syndrome [RLS]), and *secondary* insomnia that represents most patients and is due to a variety of contributing factors, including:

- *Medical* (e.g., congestive heart failure, musculoskeletal)
- *Psychiatric* (e.g., depression, anxiety)
- *Pharmacological* (e.g., prescribed or OTC medications, substances of abuse, caffeine, nicotine)
- *Other sleep disorders* (e.g., sleep apnea, restless legs syndrome, periodic limb movement disorders)

Although treating the underlying problem may resolve secondary insomnia, often both problems must be addressed to achieve the optimal outcome (e.g., antidepressant plus a sedative-hypnotic [SH] for major depression). This approach is based in part on an increasing recognition of a bidirectional interaction between various comorbid conditions and insomnia. For example, although insomnia is a frequent symptom of depression there is also evidence that insomnia increases the risk for developing depression. Table 6-2 lists the most common agents used for the treatment of insomnia.

Benzodiazepines. Although most evidence supports the use of SHs for acute, transient insomnia, these agents are also frequently used as chronic treatments despite more limited data. The BZD-SHs all work through the $GABA_A$ receptor–chloride ion complex, inhibiting neuronal firing. The various agents in this class differ primarily in their pharmacokinetics and the presence or absence of active metabolites. These issues often dictate such clinically relevant effects as onset of action, maintenance of effect, and carry-over adverse effects (e.g., EDS).

Nonbenzodiazepines. More recently, alternate agents that more specifically agonize the $GABA_A$ α subunit (i.e., BZ-1) have become available. These drugs are approved for sleep-onset insomnia

TABLE 6-2	Medications for Treatment of Insomnia	
Class/Generic Name	**Common Trade Name**	**Usual Daily Dose Range (mg/d)**
Benzodiazepines		
Long-acting		
Flurazepam	Dalmane	15–45
Quazepam	Doral	7.5–15
Intermediate acting		
Estazolam	Prosom	0.5–2
Temazepam	Restoril	15–45
Short acting		
Triazolam	Halcion	0.125–0.25
Nonbenzodiazepines		
Zolpidem	Ambien	5–20
Zolpidem CR	Ambien CR	6.25–12.5
Zaleplon	Sonata	5–20
Eszopiclone	Lunesta	2–3
Melatonin receptor agonists		
Remelteon	Rozerem	8–16
Natural remedies		
Melatonin		0.3–2
Valerian		400–900

(Adapted from Janicak PG, Davis JM, Preskorn SH, et al. *Principles and Practices of Psychopharmacotherapy*, 4th ed. Philadelphia: Lippincott Williams & Wilkins; 2006.)

and/or sleep maintenance (depending on which agent or formulation). In general, their greater pharmacodynamic specificity, lack of impact on sleep architecture, pharmacokinetics, and lower risk for drug–drug interactions make them a safer choice over the BZDs-SHs.

Melatonin Receptor Agonists. Ramelteon is a melatonin receptor agonist approved for sleep-onset insomnia. Its novel mechanism of action (i.e., affects melatonin receptors in the superchiasmatic nucleus) also suggests a potential use for circadian regulation.

Other Agents. In addition to approved drugs, several other classes of psychotropics and nonpsychotropics are often used clinically to treat sleep disorders, including:

- Antidepressants (e.g., trazodone)
- Antipsychotics (e.g., quetiapine)
- Antiepileptics (e.g., gabapentin, clonazepam)
- Antihistamines (e.g., diphenhydramine)
- Antihypertensives (e.g., clonidine in the pediatric population)
- Neutraceuticals (e.g., melatonin, valerian)

Although these agents may benefit sleep through various mechanisms, none of them have been sufficiently studied to ascertain their risk–benefit ratios for the treatment of insomnia.

Adverse Effects of Sedative-Hypnotics. Some of the more common adverse effects associated with the BZD-SHs, include:

- Excessive daytime *sedation* (particularly with longer-acting agents in older patients)
- *Cognitive* impairment (e.g., amnesia)
- *Motor* incoordination (e.g., particularly when combined with alcohol)
- *Respiratory* depression
- *Tolerance, dependence,* and *abuse*
- *Rebound insomnia* on withdrawal

The most common adverse effect with *non–BDZ*-SHs, include:

- *Headache* for all
- *Dryness of mouth* and *unpleasant taste* with eszopiclone
- *Fatigue* and *nausea* with zolpidem
- *Drowsiness* and *dizziness* with zolpidem and zolpidem CR
- *Fatigue* and *dizziness* with ramelteon

More recently, *sleep-related complex behaviors* have also been reported with agents such as zolpidem.

Other psychotropic and nonpsychotropic agents also carry specific risks for adverse events (AEs), including:

- *Priapism* with trazodone
- *Extrapyramidal side effects* (*EPS*) with antipsychotics

- *EDS* with antiepileptic drugs (AEDs)
- *Anticholinergic* effects with diphenhydramine
- *Hypotension* with clonidine
- Potential adverse *drug interactions* with valerian

Sleep-Related Breathing Disorders. The general approach to treating OSA is to encourage *weight loss*. BZDs are to be avoided because of their potential to further compromise respiratory function.

Narcolepsy. The treatment of choice is *sodium oxybate* with *stimulants* such as modafinil used to augment its efficacy. *Antidepressants* may also improve cataplexy (i.e., sudden muscle weakness especially with strong emotional reactions) often associated with this disorder. Table 6-3 lists the most common agents used to treat this condition.

Restless Legs Syndrome and Periodic Limb Movement Disorder. Although these disorders are related, they differ in their presentations and the ability to diagnose them with polysomnography. However, both are benefited by *dopamine agonists* such as ropinirole.

Circadian Rhythm Disorder. Patients with advanced or delayed phase syndromes can benefit from *fixed wake times* as well as *regular daytime and nighttime routines* to help reinforce the phase shift. *Ramelteon* and *melatonin* may also be helpful.

Device-Based Therapies for Sleep Disorders

The general approach to treating OSA is the use of *continuous positive airway pressure* (CPAP) in more severe cases. Soft tissue and/or maxillary-mandibular *surgical procedures* may also benefit patients not helped by or intolerant of CPAP.

Patients with circadian rhythm disorder and advanced or delayed phase syndromes can benefit from *bright light phototherapy* to adjust their biological clock.

Psychotherapy for Sleep Disorders

CBT for insomnia is as effective as SHs in the short term and more effective in the long term.[1-3] This conclusion is based on the results of numerous controlled trials comparing CBT with

TABLE 6-3	Medications for Treatment of Narcolepsy	
Class/Generic Name	Common Trade Name	Usual Daily Dose Range (mg/d)
Treatments for cataplexy		
■ Antidepressants		
■ Fluoxetine	Prozac	60 mg/d
■ Venlafaxine	Effexor	75–375 mg/d
■ Imipramine	Tofranil	25–100 mg/d
■ Protriptyline	Vivactyl	10–40 mg/d
■ Sodium oxybate	Xyrem	3–9 g/d
Treatments for excessive daytime sleepiness (EDS)		
■ Stimulants		
■ Modafinil	Provigil	200–400 mg/d
■ Dextroamphetamine	Dexedrine	5–60 mg/d
■ Methylphenidate	Ritalin	5–60 mg/d
■ Sodium oxybate	Xyrem	4.5–9 g/d
■ Combinations		
■ Sodium oxybate plus modafinil for long-term management		

pharmacotherapy, placebo, or reduced components of the entire CBT protocol (e.g., relaxation training). Components of CBT for insomnia include:

- Stimulus control
- Sleep restriction
- Sleep hygiene
- Relaxation training
- Cognitive therapy (CT)

Stimulus control is typically recommended as the initial treatment of sleep onset and maintenance problems. The focus of this intervention is to reinforce the association between the bed or bedroom and sleep. The instructions include:

- Go to sleep only when you are ready to sleep
- Avoid any other behaviors (e.g., eating, watching television) beside sleep and sex in the bedroom
- If you are awake for >15 minutes, get out of bed
- Return to bed only when you are sleepy
- Maintain a fixed wake and sleep cycle, 7 days a week

The aim is to have the patient begin to reassociate sleep with the bed and bedroom.

Sleep restriction is an optional component to CBT for insomnia, primarily because it has not been studied independently. The focus of this component is to restrict the time patients spend in bed to an amount equal to their average time in bed sleeping. Many patients, in an attempt to get more sleep, spend significant amounts of time lying in bed trying to sleep. Therefore, sleep restriction alters that habit so that patients are in bed only for the amount of time that they have been getting sleep. Sleep logs will help the clinician determine how much sleep a patient is actually getting a night. On the basis of that number, but no less than 4.5 hours, the clinician and patient will restrict the sleep to that amount. This is difficult for the patient but it is an important step to consolidating sleep time.

Sleep hygiene focuses on educating patients about healthy sleep habits that facilitate their compliance with the other components. Altering sleep habits can be very difficult. Imagine no longer reading or watching television in bed, habits almost universal in many cultures. If patients understand why they need to make such changes, they are more likely to try. Table 6-4 lists the techniques that are recommended to improve sleep.

Relaxation training is a second-line treatment that can be helpful for patients who are very tense or describe hypervigilance as their usual physical state. This component includes teaching patients progressive muscle relaxation, imagery, diaphragmatic breathing, and other relaxation techniques.

Although these interventions are identified as CBT, many of the components are behavioral in nature. This again reflects some of the difficulty separating cognitive and behavioral elements of an intervention. For many patients, however, the *cognitive restructuring or CT* component is very important. After months of

TABLE 6-4	*Sleep Hygiene Techniques*

Should

- Maintain a regular sleep–wake schedule
- Regularly exercise in morning/afternoon (at least 3 h before bedtime)
- Increase exposure to bright light during the day
- Use relaxing techniques close to bedtime
  - Warm bath

Should avoid

- Daytime
  - Napping
  - Excessive use of caffeine or nicotine
- 4–6 h before bedtime
  - Caffeine
- 3–4 hours before bedtime
  - Exercise
- Close to bedtime
  - Alcohol
  - Heavy meals (have a light snack if hungry)
  - Extra liquids
- While in bed
  - Noise, light, or uncomfortable temperatures
  - Activities other than sleep or sex
  - Watching the clock
  - Smoking when you wake up

not getting adequate rest, many patients begin to worry, predict failure, and imagine catastrophic results from another sleepless night. The CT component focuses on challenging such beliefs and reducing anxious thoughts.

> Mr. Z initiated the sleep hygiene techniques with some difficulty. He found it very hard to eliminate watching television in bed and it was even more of a struggle to maintain the same wake time on the weekends. Because the patient was getting approximately 5.5 hours of sleep, based on his sleep logs, we began to restrict his time in bed to this duration. We also dealt with his heightened anxiety as he neared the time to go to bed. He had thoughts he was going to be awake all night and this was never going to improve.

Combined Psychotherapy and Pharmacotherapy for Sleep Disorders

There is little controlled trial data looking at the sequencing or combining of psychotherapy and pharmacotherapy for the various sleep disorders. Jacobs et al.[4] compared CBT and pharmacotherapy and found that the combination of CBT and SHs in the treatment of insomnia was no better than CBT alone. Although the data clearly supports CBT as the primary first-line treatment approach, patients will likely be prescribed a sleep aid and it is often best to first introduce CBT with the goal of tapering medications to develop an effective long-term strategy. Perlis et al.[5] in their session-by-session guide propose that CBT for insomnia is most effective if the medications are discontinued before CBT is initiated. If not feasible, they recommend collaborating with the prescribing physician to phase out medication to better ensure the long-term effectiveness of CBT as a stand-alone treatment.

Introducing Combined Treatment

We discussed with Mr. Z the potential value of sleep medication in the short term and also that eventually he would need a more viable long-term sleep stabilizing strategy. This was in recognition of the reccurring nature of his sleep disturbance and his potential vulnerability to these problems under stress. It was proposed that we could work together to provide him with additional coping strategies. In collaboration with his PCP, we developed a 4-week plan to reduce the dose of zolpidem by half each week, thereby limiting the negative effects of withdrawal.

If the interventions are provided by two clinicians, it is very important to communicate and maintain a consistent treatment plan.

Questions to ask the psychotherapist
- *What techniques have been most effective for this patient?*
- *In what time frame can I begin to taper his medication?*
- *Does it make sense to reintroduce medication on an intermittent basis in combination with the CBT techniques?*

Questions to ask the pharmacotherapist
- *What is your plan for the medication?*
- *Are there any contraindications to CBT for insomnia (e.g., sleep restriction) with this patient?*
- *What medication side effects should I monitor?*

CLINICAL RECOMMENDATIONS

For the management of insomnia, we first recommend ruling out any *potential underlying condition* (e.g., OSA, RLS) and treating such problems to resolution. If no cause is identified or the insomnia persists, then the various *cognitive behavioral techniques* are the next approach. With sleep–wake problems, bright light phototherapy with or without CBT may be the initial approach. If CBT is insufficient or unavailable, then short-term use of a *non-BDZ or BZD-SH* is appropriate. We would suggest, however, avoiding their use in patients with OSA because these agents may further suppress the respiratory drive. If SHs are necessary for longer periods, we recommend eszoplicone, zolpidem CR, and possibly ramelteon. Finally, coordinating the use of a SH with CBT may allow for the slow reduction and cessation of the SH. The object is to use CBT alone for maintenance treatment.

For the management of narcolepsy, *sodium oxybate* is the recommended first-line treatment. With insufficient response, the addition of *modafinil* or an alternate stimulant may improve efficacy. For patients with more significant cataplexy, an *antidepressant* (selective serotonin reuptake inhibitor [SSRI] or tricyclic antidepressant [TCA]) combined with sodium oxybate may improve overall functioning.

CBT and other sleep hygiene strategies are outlined in several textbooks that are helpful to clinicians.[5,6] In addition, there are several self-help books available but the efficacy of self-help treatments for insomnia are unknown.[7]

Mr. Z after 4 weeks of treatment, in collaboration with his PCP, weaned himself from the zolpidem. Gradually, with time and practice the sleep hygiene techniques became more regular habits. After setting a sleep–wake cycle to include 5.5 hours of sleep, we continued to monitor his quality of sleep. As the patient reached the level of sleeping for 90% of the time spent in bed, the duration was increased by 15 minutes. We continued to incrementally increase his time in bed over the next few weeks. In addition, with the use of relaxation techniques and cognitive restructuring, his anxiety decreased and the frequency of his negative thoughts about the future were significantly reduced. Eventually Mr. Z was able to fall asleep within 15 minutes and slept on average 7 hours, only wakening a few minutes each night.

Figures 6-1 and 6-2 outline the approaches we would recommend for insomnia and narcolepsy.

Learning points

- Sleep disorders are common in the general population (i.e., ~70 million will experience difficulty).
- Treatment approaches vary depending on the types of disorders (e.g., insomnia vs. hypersomnia).
- Such varied approaches as medication, CBT, bright light phototherapy, CPAP, and surgical procedures may all play a role depending on the specific disorder.
- Temporarily incorporating the biological treatment approach with CBT may benefit the patient in the long term.

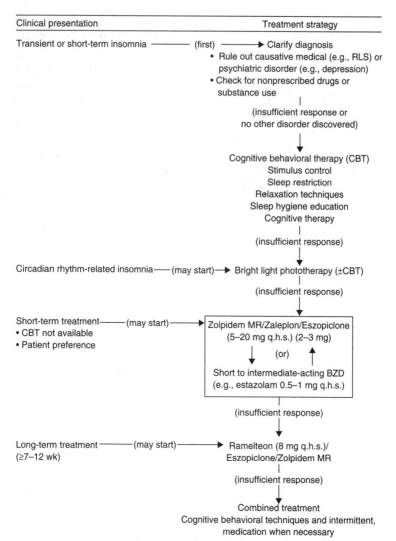

FIGURE 6-1 ■ Treatment strategy for insomnia. RLS, restless leg syndrome; BZD, benzodiazepines. (Adapted from Janicak PG, Davis JM, Preskorn SH, et al. *Principles and Practice of Psychopharmacotherapy*, 4th ed. Philadelphia: Lippincott Williams & Wilkins; 2006:492.)

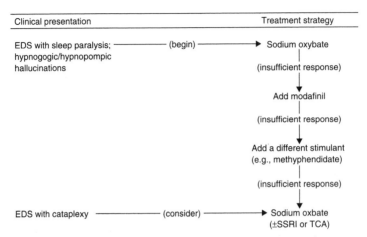

Clinical presentation	Treatment strategy

EDS with sleep paralysis; ——— (begin) ———▶ Sodium oxybate
hypnogogic/hypnopompic
hallucinations   (insufficient response)

Add modafinil

(insufficient response)

Add a different stimulant
(e.g., methyphendidate)

(insufficient response)

EDS with cataplexy ——————— (consider) ———▶ Sodium oxbate
(±SSRI or TCA)

FIGURE 6-2 ▧ Treatment strategy for narcolepsy with excessive daytime sleepiness. EDS, excessive daytime sleepiness; SSRI, selective serotonin reuptake inhibitor; TCA, tricyclic antidepressant.

REFERENCES

1. Smith MT, Perlis ML, Park A, et al. Comparative meta-analysis of pharmacotherapy and behavior therapy for persistent insomniacs? *Am J psychiatry.* 2002;159:5–11.
2. Sibler MH. Chronic Insomnia. *N Engl J Med.* 2005;353:803–810.
3. Sivertsen B, Omvik S, Pallesen S, et al. Cognitive behavioral therapy versus zopiclone for treatment of chronic primary insomnia in older adults. A randomized controlled trial. *JAMA.* 2006;295(24): 2851–2858.
4. Jacobs GD, Pace-Schott EF, Stickgold R, et al. Cognitive behavioral therapy and pharmacotherapy for insomnia a randomized controlled trial and direct comparison. *Arch Intern Med.* 2004;164: 1888–1896.
5. Perlis ML, Jungquist C, Smithe MT, et al. *Cognitive behavioral treatment of insomnia: a session by session guide.* New York: Springer; 2005.
6. Morin CM, Espie CA. *Insomnia: a clinician's guide to assessment and treatment.* New York: Guilford Press; 2003.
7. Espie A. *Overcoming insomnia and sleep problems.* New York: New York University Press; 2006.

SUGGESTED READINGS

American Psychiatric Association. *Diagnostic and statistical manual of mental disorders*, 4th ed. Text Revision. Washington, DC: 2000.

Edinger JD, Means MK. Cognitive behavioral therapy for primary insomnia. *Clin Psychol Rev.* 2005;25(5):539–558.

Edinger JD, Wohlgemuth WK, Radtke RA, et al. Cognitive behavioral therapy for treatment of chronic primary insomnia: A randomized controlled trial. *JAMA.* 2001;285(14):1856–1864.

Foley D, Ancoli-Israel S, Britz P, et al. Sleep disturbances and chronic disease in older adults: Results of the 2003 National Sleep Foundation Sleep in America Survey. *J Psychosom Res.* 2004;56(5):497–502.

Gordon ML, Doghramji PR, Lieberman JA III. Stay awake! Understanding, diagnosing and successfully managing narcolepsy. *Curr Psychiatry.* 2007;S3–S16.

Janicak PG, Davis JM, Preskorn SH, et al. *Principles and practice of psychopharmacotherapy*, 4th ed. Philadelphia: Lippincott Williams & Wilkins; 2006.

Leshner A. National Institutes of Health State of the Science Conference statement on manifestations and management of chronic insomnia in adults, June 13–15, 2005. *Sleep.* 2005;28(9):1049–1057.

Mendelson W. A review of the evidence for the efficacy and safety of trazodone in insomnia. *J Clin Psychiatry.* 2005;66(4):469–476.

National Heart, Lung, and Blood Institute, Working Group on Insomnia. Insomnia: Assessment and management in primary care. *Am Fam Physician.* 1999;59(11):3029–3038.

Nofzinger EA, Buysse DJ, Germain A, et al. Functional neuroimaging evidence for hyperarousal in insomnia. *Am J Psychiatry.* 2004;161(11): 2126–2128.

Trenkwalder C, Garcia-Borreguero D, Montagna P, et al. Ropinirole in the treatment of restless legs syndrome: Results from the TREAT RLS 1 study, a 12 week, randomised; placebo controlled study in 10 European countries. *J Neurol Neurosurg Psychiatry.* 2004;75(1): 92–97.

Schizophrenia

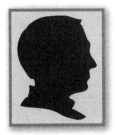

Mr. Q

Mr. Q is a 23-year-old, single male who presented with paranoid delusions and auditory hallucinations. He had three previous episodes of psychosis beginning at age 19 when he was first hospitalized. Mr. Q describes that others are out to get him but does not know why. He also reports that when he leaves home, people are paying special attention to him and following him. He hears a voice warning of danger and the need to protect himself. Mr. Q has been unable to finish college and spends most of his time in the basement of the family home. He reports enjoying watching television but has no friends or social contacts. The family tends to leave him alone but brings dinner in the evenings. The family also reports that he is not compliant with medications and in the last few weeks has become increasingly agitated, paranoid, and withdrawn.

Schizophrenia is a severe, chronic, psychotic disorder. The lifetime prevalence worldwide is often quoted as 1%, but may vary slightly based on demographics such as economic class and gender. Although there is an equal distribution between men and women, men develop clinical symptoms approximately 6 years earlier. Onset is usually during adolescence and early adulthood. This disorder is characterized by various *symptom complexes*, which include the following:

- *Positive* (e.g., hallucinations, delusions)
- *Negative* or deficit (e.g., isolation, amotivation)
- *Cognitive* (e.g., verbal and nonverbal working memory, executive functioning, verbal and visual learning)
- *Mood* (e.g., dysphoric, suicidal ideation)

These symptoms may vary over time with most individuals experiencing a gradual deterioration in their ability to function. Negative and cognitive symptoms are the most disabling and less amenable to treatment. In addition, these patients are plagued by high rates of suicide and comorbidity with other psychiatric and medical disorders. As a result, their life expectancies are substantially shortened compared to the general population.

Mr. Q meets criteria for schizophrenia, paranoid type. He has delusions and hallucinations but denies any affective component. He is withdrawn and has no interest in social interactions. He experienced a significant decrease in functioning over the last 4 years and is now completely inactive.

DIFFERENTIAL DIAGNOSIS

The differential diagnosis of schizophrenia includes a variety of conditions that may present with psychotic symptoms. Some of the more common considerations are:

- *Schizoaffective* disorder
- *Delusional* disorder
- *Mood* disorders with psychosis (e.g., acute mania with delusions)
- *Drug-induced* psychotic episodes (e.g., phencyclidine intoxication)
- *Psychosis* secondary to a nonpsychiatric medical condition (e.g., dementia with psychosis)

NEUROBIOLOGY

The development of clinical symptoms involves a complex interaction between biological predisposition (e.g., genetics) and environmental stressors (e.g., viral infection) occurring during critical developmental periods (e.g., fetal, neonatal, puberty). These abnormal *neurodevelopmental* events are further exacerbated by subsequent *neurodegenerative* processes as evidenced by imaging studies, which demonstrate:

- *Structural* brain volume changes
- Changes in *functional* activity in relevant neurocircuits
- Altered central nervous system (CNS) *blood flow* and *glucose metabolism*
- *Biochemical* alterations in related CNS regions

For example, progressive reductions in *frontal lobe gray and white matter* correlate with functional impairment in schizophrenia. Further, lower *hippocampal volumes* are found in both patients and their nonpsychotic first-degree relatives. In addition, functional deficits in *cortical and subcortical areas* are observed in those patients who are medication-free, first-episode schizophrenia and may also appear in unaffected siblings. Clinical issues often associated with *reduced cortical volume* and *enlarged ventricles* include:

- Soft *neurologic* signs
- Poorer *response* to treatment
- Worse *prognosis*

TREATMENT OF SCHIZOPHRENIA

Ideally, early detection and prevention represent the optimal strategy for schizophrenia and other psychotic disorders. In this context, certain factors may improve prediction in younger individuals,[1] including:

- *Genetic risk* with recent *functional deterioration*
- Higher levels of *unusual thought content*
- Higher levels of *suspicion/paranoia*
- Greater *social impairment*
- History of *substance abuse*

Although work continues on earlier interventions to preclude a full episode, most patients are first treated after they meet full criteria for schizophrenia.

Pharmacotherapy for Schizophrenia

The use of *antipsychotics* is the primary mode of treatment to control acute exacerbations, reduce relapse rates, and prevent recurrence.[2] Although both first-generation antipsychotics (FGAs) and second-generation antipsychotics (SGAs) are effective for positive symptoms, SGAs arguably produce additional benefit in negative, cognitive, and mood symptoms compared to their first-generation counterparts. For example, clozapine is the only antipsychotic approved by the U.S. Food and Drug Administration (FDA) for management of suicidal symptoms in patients with schizophrenia or schizoaffective disorder. The SGAs have also demonstrated a more robust effect then placebo or FGAs in reducing relapse rates. These results, however, were derived from randomized, placebo, or active comparator-controlled trials and may not readily translate into more real-world conditions as evidenced by the results of the National Institute of Mental Health (NIMH)–sponsored Clinical Antipsychotic Trials of Intervention Effectiveness (CATIE) Study.[3]

Therefore, the choice of antipsychotic often depends on the safety and tolerability profile of a specific agent matched to an individual's proclivity for developing certain complications (e.g., a personal or family history of diabetes). Tables 7-1 and 7-2 list the various classes of antipsychotics and their common adverse effect profiles.

Mr. Q was prescribed an oral antipsychotic (risperidone 4 mg per day) but the family reported that he was not compliant. Therefore, risperidone long-acting injectable formulation was initiated at 25 mg biweekly.

Device-Based Therapies for Schizophrenia

Electroconvulsive Therapy. Although medication remains the primary treatment strategy for schizophrenia, electroconvulsive therapy (ECT), usually in combination with an antipsychotic, has demonstrated acute benefit, particularly in patients with severe mood symptoms, suicidal behavior, or catatonia.[4] Examples of other situations where ECT may be considered include patients refractory to clozapine (using ECT for augmentation) and patients who have recently experienced an episode of neuroleptic malignant syndrome (NMS) secondary to their antipsychotic medication (using ECT as an alternative).[5,6]

Transcranial Magnetic Stimulation. Preliminary evidence demonstrates the potential efficacy of transcranial magnetic stimulation (TMS) for positive symptoms such as auditory hallucinations.[7] The evidence that TMS benefits negative symptoms is less compelling. Presently, there is a need to clarify and optimize TMS' delivery for specific psychotic symptoms to determine its utility in schizophrenia.[8]

Psychotherapy for Schizophrenia

Unfortunately, the complexity of symptoms manifested in schizophrenia makes the psychotherapy of choice unclear. Numerous studies have examined various approaches, always as adjuncts to medication. Many of these adjunctive therapies reduced relapse, increased functioning, increased social skills, and reduced family stress. The decision as to which patient is best suited for a specific treatment, however, depends on the presenting symptoms, course of illness, and social situation. Several therapeutic approaches are reported to be efficacious, including:

- *Cognitive* behavioral therapy for psychosis (CBTp)
- *Family* therapy
- *Social* skills training
- *Vocational* rehabilitation/*occupational* skills training/supported *employment*
- Cognitive *remediation*/cognitive *enhancement* therapy/*neurocognitive* therapy

CBTp was developed in the United Kingdom and reported to improve positive symptoms of schizophrenia.[9] The best benefit with CBTp appears to be in chronic, partially remitted patients, with less support for benefit in acutely ill patients. In a meta-analysis of seven randomized controlled trials of CBT for delusions and hallucinations, however, Gould et al.[10] found large effect sizes with five of the seven studies evidencing significant symptom reduction before and after CBT treatment. This approach involves a careful case formulation to determine each individual's experiences, focusing on one's thoughts, behavior, and emotional responses in the context of their environment. The aim is to develop alternate coping strategies.

Family therapy incorporates several interventions including education, support, development of coping mechanisms, and communication training. Multiple studies report that this approach reduces relapse rates.

Social skills training breaks down complex social skills into learnable steps using practice and role modeling. This training is effective with evidence that the newly developed skills also generalize to real-world interactions.

Vocational rehabilitation is a complex job training program that matches the patient's level of functioning with a specific occupation. These programs enhance the patients' skills and

Class/Generic Name	Common Trade Name	Usual Daily Dose Range
TABLE 7-1 *Medications for Treatment of Schizophrenia*		
First-Generation Antipsychotics		
Phenothiazines		
Aliphatics		
Chlorpromazine	Thorazine	100–1,000
Promazine	Sparine	25–1,000
Triflupromazine	Vesprin	20–150
Piperidines		
Thioridazine	Mellaril	30–800
Mesoridazine	Serentil	20–200
Piperacetazine	Quide	20–160
Piperazines		
Trifluoperazine	Stelazine	2–60
Fluphenazine	Prolixin	5–40
Perphenazine	Trilafon	2–60
Acetophenazine	Tindal	40–80
Prochlorperazine	Compazine	15–125
Thioxanthenes		
Thiothixene	Navane	6–60
Chlorprothixene	Taractan	10–600
Dibenzoxazepines		
Loxapine	Loxitane	20–250
Butyrophenones		
Haloperidol	Haldol	3–20
Droperidol	Inapsin	[a]2.5–10
Diphenylbutylpiperidines		
Pimozide	Orap	1–10
Dihyproindolones		
Molindone	Moban	15–225

TABLE 7-1	Medications for Treatment of Schizophrenia (continued)	
Class/Generic Name	Common Trade Name	Usual Daily Dose Range
Second-Generation Antipsychotics		
Dibenzodiazepines		
Clozapine	Clozaril	100–900
Benzisoxazoles		
Risperidone	Risperdal	2–8
Risperidone microspheres	Risperdal Consta	25–50 biweekly
Paliperidone ER	Invega	3–12
Thienobenzodiazepines		
Olanzapine	Zyprexa	5–20
Dibenzothiazepines		
Quetiapine	Seroquel	75–800
Benzisothiazolyls		
Ziprasidone	Geodon	40–160
Quinolinoles		
Aripiprazole	Abilify	5–30

[a]Administered intramuscularly.
(Adapted from Janicak PG, Davis JM, Preskorn SH, et al. *Principles and Practice of Psychopharmacotherapy*, 4th ed. Philadelphia: Lippincott Williams & Wilkins; 2006.)

prepare them for work. Techniques include on-site coaching and support which are associated with significant improvement in employment and job retention.

Cognitive remediation focuses on the neurocognitive impairments associated with schizophrenia. Treatment involves practice exercises and drills targeting verbal and visual memory, attention, and cognitive flexibility. This approach has been shown to improve neurocognition, reduce symptoms, and improve overall functioning and work performance.[11,12]

TABLE 7-2	Adverse Effects of Antipsychotics[a]							
	HPDL	CLOZ	RISP	OLZ	QTP	ZIP	ARIP	PALI
Neurologic	+++	0	+	0/+	0	0/+	0/+	+
Weight gain/endocrine	+	+++	++	+++	++	0/+	0	++
Anticholinergic	0	+++	0/+	+/++	0/+	0/+	0	0/+
Hematologic	0	+++	0	0	0	0	0	0
Cardiovascular	+	0/+	+	+	+	++	0	+
Prolactin	++	0/+	+++	0/+	0/+	0/+	0	+++
Sedation	+	+++	+	+/++	++	++	+	+

[a]At appropriate doses, 0 = none; + = mild; ++ = moderate; +++ = substantial.
HPDL, haloperidol; CLOZ, clozapine; RISP, risperidone; OLZ, olanzapine; QTP, quetiapine; ZIP, ziprasidone; ARIP, aripiprazole; PALI, paliperidone ER. (Adapted from Masand PS. Handbook of psychiatry in primary care; 1998.)

In a recent meta-analysis, McGurk et al.[13] found that combining cognitive remediation with vocational rehabilitation further improved functional outcomes.

Mr. Q's significant negative symptoms and supportive family involvement led to the recommendation for family therapy and a vocational rehabilitation program. Family therapy focused on educating the family members about both the positive and negative symptoms of schizophrenia, providing support to help them accept the changes in their son as well as problem solving to more effectively increase structure to Mr. Q's day. In addition, the patient began a day hospital program with the hope of linking him to vocational training as his symptoms stabilized. Mr. Q was reluctant to attend the program, however, because he continued to feel unsafe. The dose of risperidone microspheres was increased to 37.5 mg biweekly, which helped increase his comfort level at the day hospital.

Combined Psychotherapy and Pharmacotherapy for Schizophrenia

Although antipsychotics are the mainstay of treatment, their overall impact is muted by several issues, which include:

- *Partial* or *insufficient effectiveness* for various symptoms
- *Adverse effects*
- *Low adherence* rates
- Inadequate *social support* systems

Therefore, psychotherapeutic and psychosocial interventions are frequently employed to augment the benefits experienced with medications and to promote better adherence. Increasingly, the emphasis is not only symptom reduction but also development of comprehensive strategies that lead to *functional recovery*.[14]

Introducing Combined Treatment

Medications are necessary to control acute exacerbations of psychotic symptoms but must be combined with other approaches to optimize long-term outcomes. Therefore, the early introduction of psychotherapy may prevent further deterioration and substantially improve the capacity to carry out daily activities and to achieve the goal of functional recovery.

> *Possible discussion points include:*
> - *Because medication is essential for you to continue improving, it is important that we discuss the benefits and side effects and how you can develop a strategy to stay on your medication.*
> - *In addition to your medication, there are other therapies that can help you think more clearly, feel more comfortable in social interactions, and find work that is satisfying.*
> - *We would like to include your family in treatment because we want to educate them about your illness and how they can help you improve the quality of your life.*
> - *We want to help you and your family understand how the nature of your illness impacts your ability to think, focus, and carry out even ordinary responsibilities.*
> - *There is also a specific therapy called CBT that can help you develop new strategies to cope with your symptoms.*

In the context of schizophrenia, the involvement of several providers is the norm (e.g., psychiatrist, psychologist, social worker, counselor, case manager). Therefore, open communication among these various professionals is a prerequisite for a successful treatment strategy.

Questions to ask the psychotherapist

- *Which approaches are best given the patient's degree of illness, family involvement, and community support?*
- *What is the level of neurocognitive impairment and how can we target these symptoms?*
- *What is the patient's functional level and how can we further improve it?*

Questions to ask the pharmacotherapist

- *Which approaches are best given the patients degree of illness, family involvement, and community support?*
- *How can we ensure the patient's adherence to medications?*
- *What side effects should we monitor, particularly as they negatively impact the patient's ability to think, ability to function, and overall health status?*
- *How can we minimize the potential adverse effects of an otherwise effective antipsychotic (e.g., weight gain and associated complications)?*

CLINICAL RECOMMENDATIONS

For an acute exacerbation, the immediate strategy employs an antipsychotic to rapidly control symptoms with a high risk for serious consequences (e.g., self-harm, aggressive behavior toward others, avoiding or minimizing time in the hospital). Considering the existing evidence base, clinical experience, and safety–tolerability profile, we would begin with a nonclozapine SGA. The addition of psychotherapy may also be useful in an acute exacerbation for patients who can cooperate or for families that need additional support. The primary antipsychotic agent could be augmented temporarily with a benzodiazepine or acute intramuscular formulation of certain SGAs to quickly control agitation, aggressive behaviors, and alcohol or drug withdrawal symptoms when present. If response is inadequate, trials with other SGAs (including clozapine) or an FGA may be alternative approaches. In patients with significant mood-related complications (e.g., high suicidality), the use of adjunctive antidepressants or an antiepileptic mood stabilizer may help. Alternatively, a trial with clozapine may be indicated. Long-acting injectible formulations of an SGA (e.g., risperidone microspheres) or FGA (e.g., haloperidol decanoate) may be better choices with patients who demonstrate poor response and/or poor adherence to orally administered agents. We also recommend the addition of psychotherapy to target the patient's specific needs whether it is symptom reduction, increasing social skills, or vocational rehabilitation.

In treatment refractory patients, a definitive trial of clozapine should be implemented. A course of ECT may be the most effective strategy in patients with catatonia, who are highly suicidal or refractory to medication. TMS may be an alternate approach to reduce specific symptoms (e.g., medication-resistant auditory hallucinations).

Given the high risk of relapse and recurrence in schizophrenia, indefinite maintenance therapy is usually required. During the maintenance phase, we would use ongoing psychotherapeutic approaches to enhance the benefits of medication, to increase functioning, to help improve adherence rates, and to provide education and support to both patients and their caregivers.

Mr. Q adjusted to the day program and became more involved with his family. He continued to be suspicious at times but was able to use the coping skills he learned at the day program to handle his fears. He continued on risperidone long-acting injections every 2 weeks and with family support was more consistent with taking his medications.

Figures 7-1 and 7-2 outline the strategies we would recommend for both acute and maintenance treatment.

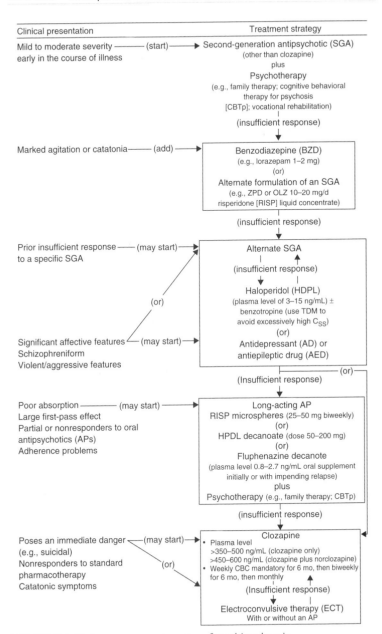

FIGURE 7-1 ■ Acute treatment strategy for schizophrenia.
ZPD, ziprasidone; OLZ, olanzapine; TDM, therapeutic drug monitoring.
(Adapted from Janicak PG, Davis JM, Preskorn SH, et al. *Principles and Practice of Psychopharmacotherapy*, 4th ed. Philadelphia: Lippincott Williams & Wilkins; 2006:116.)

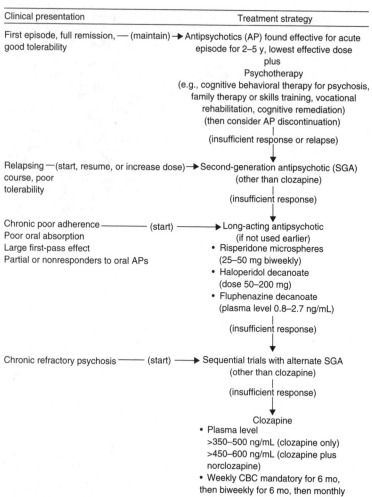

FIGURE 7-2 ■ Maintenance treatment strategy for schizophrenia. (Adapted from Janicak PG, Davis JM, Preskorn SH, et al. *Principles and Practice of Psychopharmacotherapy*, 4th ed. Philadelphia: Lippincott Williams & Wilkins; 2006.)

Learning points

- Schizophrenia is a chronic psychotic condition that requires lifelong treatment.

- Antipsychotics vary in terms of safety and tolerability issues and arguably in certain efficacy issues.
- Psychotherapeutic interventions can significantly enhance improvement and facilitate functional recovery in these patients.
- Device-based treatments such as ECT may be helpful in certain presentations.

REFERENCES

1. Cannon TD, Cadenhead K, Cornblatt B, et al. Prediction of psychosis in youth at high clinical risk: A multisite longitudinal study in North America. *Arch Gen Psychiatry.* 2008;65(1):28–37.

2. Janicak PG, Davis JM, Preskorn SH, et al. *Principles and practice of psychopharmacotherapy,* 4th ed. Philadelphia: Lippincott Williams & Wilkins; 2006.

3. Lieberman JA, Stroup TS, McEvoy JP, et al. Clinical Antipsychotic Trials of Intervention Effectiveness (CATIE) Investigators. Effectiveness of antipsychotic drugs in patients with chronic schizophrenia. *N Engl J Med.* 2005;353(12):1209–1223.

4. Tharyan P, Adams CE. Electroconvulsive therapy for schizophrenia. *Cochrane Database Syst Rev.* 2005;2:CD000076.

5. Braga RJ, Petrides G. The combined use of electroconvulsive therapy and antipsychotics in patients with schizophrenia. *J ECT.* 2005;21(2): 75–83.

6. Pierce K, Flynn P, Caudle M, et al. Electroconvulsive therapy (ECT): Current clinical standards. *Psychopharm Rev.* 2008;43(5):35–42.

7. Aleman A, Sommer IE, Kahn RS. Efficacy of slow repetitive transcranial magnetic stimulation in the treatment of resistant auditory hallucinations in schizophrenia: A meta-analysis. *J Clin Psychiatry.* 2007; 68(3):416–421.

8. Stanford AD, Sharif Z, Corcoran C, et al. rTMS strategies for the study and treatment of schizophrenia: A review. *Int J Neuropsychopharmacol.* 2008;1–14; (Epub ahead of print).

9. Zimmerman G, Favrod J, Trieu VH, et al. The effect of cognitive behavioral treatment on the positive symptoms of schizophrenia spectrum disorders: A meta-analysis. *Schizophr Res.* 2005;77(1): 1–9.

10. Gould RA, Mueser KT, Bolton E, et al. Cognitive therapy for psychosis in schizophrenia: An effect size analysis. *Schizophr Res.* 2001; 48(2-3):335–342.

11. Twamley EW, Jeste DV, Bellack AS. A review of cognitive training in schizophrenia. *Schizophr Bull.* 2004;29(2):359–382.

12. Lindenmayer JP, McGurk SR, Mueser KT, et al. A randomized controlled trial of cognitive remediation among inpatients with persistent mental illness. *Psychiatr Serv.* 2008;59(3):241–247.
13. McGurk AR, Twamley EW, Sitzer DI, et al. A meta-analysis of cognitive remediation in schizophrenia. *Am J Psychiatry.* 2007;164(12): 1791–1801.
14. Green MF, Nuechterlein KH, Kern RS, et al. Functional co-primary measures for clinical trials in schizophrenia: Results from the MATRICS psychometric and standardization study. *Am J Psychiatry.* 2008;165(2):221–228.

SUGGESTED READINGS

Fisher JR, O'Donohue WT, eds. *Practitioner's guide to evidence-based psychotherapy.* New York, NY: Springer; 2006.
Hunt GE, Bergen J, Bashir M. Medication compliance and comorbid substance abuse in schizophrenia: Impact on community survival 4 years after a relapse. *Schizophr Res.* 2002;54(3):253–264.
Lam DH, Watkins ER, Hayward P, et al. A randomized controlled study of cognitive therapy for relapse prevention for bipolar affective disorder: Outcome of the first year. *Arch Gen Psychiatry.* 2003;60(2): 145–152.
Lehman AF, Lieberman JA, Dixon LB, et al. American Psychiatric Association; Steering Committee on Practice Guidelines. Practice guidelines for the treatment of patients with schizophrenia, second edition. *Am J Psychiatry.* 2004;161(Suppl 2):1–56.
Lenroot R, Bustillo JR, Lauriello AJ, et al. Integrated treatment of schizophrenia. *Psychiatr Serv.* 2003;54(11):1499–1507.
Masand PS. *Handbook of psychiatry in primary care;* 1998.
McEvoy JP. Risk versus benefits of different types of long-acting injectable antipsychotics. *J Clin Psychiatry.* 2006;67(Suppl 5):15–18.
Olfson M, Marcus SC, Wilk J, et al. Awareness of illness and nonadherence to antipsychotic medications among persons with schizophrenia. *Psychiatr Serv.* 2006;57(2):205–211.
Tarrier N, Lewis S, Haddock G, et al. Cognitive-behavioral therapy in first-episode and early schizophrenia. 18-month follow-up of a randomized controlled trial. *Br J Psychiatry.* 2004;184:231–239.

Bipolar Disorder

LEARNING OBJECTIVES

The reader will be able to:

1. Understand the differences and relationship between pharmacotherapy, device-based therapies, and psychotherapy for the treatment of bipolar disorder (BPD).
2. Develop strategies for combined or sequenced treatment approaches for BPD.
3. Enhance skills to negotiate these treatment approaches with patients.

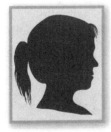

Ms. R

Ms. R is a 32-year-old, married woman who presented with irritable mood, agitation, pressured speech, and a decreased need for sleep over the last 3 weeks. She has two children (ages 3 years and 9 months). Ms. R had several previous depressive and manic episodes and two hospitalizations. Her husband brought her for treatment as he noticed a significant increase in symptoms over the last week.

Bipolar disorder (BPD) is characterized by chronic, recurrent, disabling mood symptoms further complicated by high rates

115

of suicide, substance use, comorbid psychiatric disorders, and mortality. All contribute to the lower life expectancy seen in this condition. The US lifetime prevalence rate of bipolar I disorder is estimated to be 1.3%. When bipolar II and other more subtle forms of the illness (e.g., cyclothymic disorder) are included, the prevalence rate may be as high as 3.7%. There is an equal distribution among ethnic groups and between men and women. The onset of this disorder is usually before the age of 20 peaking between the ages of 15 to 19, but a definitive diagnosis is often delayed by several years. BPD produces substantial disability and functional impairment in work, leisure, and interpersonal activities, both during and between mood episodes.

Mania/hypomania, depression, or *their combination* (i.e., mixed states) are the primary mood symptoms. Bipolar I disorder includes full mania and full depression, whereas bipolar II disorder involves hypomania and full depression. Associated symptoms of mania/hypomania may include hyperactivity, pressured speech, flight of ideas, inflated self-esteem, decreased need for sleep, distractibility, and excessive involvement in activities that have a high potential for painful consequences. The course of illness can vary from only a few episodes to a more virulent pattern characterized by multiple episodes over short periods of time (e.g., rapid cycling that involves four or more episodes per year). Of note, depression is often the heralding symptom and patients usually experience more time depressed than manic/hypomanic over the course of their illness. More severe episodes can present with psychotic features and impulsive destructive behavior. For example, the suicide rate for BPD is approximately 10% in untreated patients and approximately 25% attempt suicide at some point. The risk for suicide is greatest during a depressed or mixed symptom episode.

Ms. R was first diagnosed with BPD at age 20. At that time, she experienced a full manic episode spending all her savings, sleeping only 2 to 3 hours a night, and feeling very energized and upbeat. Owing to the severity of her symptoms she was hospitalized. Since then, Ms. R has experienced two more manic episodes as well as several episodes of depression. For the last 7 years she has been stable, and during this time was married and started a family.

DIFFERENTIAL DIAGNOSIS

BPD is often mistaken for other conditions (e.g., unipolar depression, schizophrenia, attention deficit hyperactivity disorder [ADHD]). This can substantially delay accurate diagnosis and implementation of appropriate treatment. Further, other comorbid conditions are common (e.g., substance abuse) and can also impede proper diagnosis.

Secondary mania can be precipitated by a variety of medical conditions (e.g., hyperthyroidism, complex partial seizures), medications (e.g., steroids, tricyclic antidepressants), or drug intoxication/withdrawal (e.g., amphetamines, cocaine).

Substance and alcohol abuse or dependence frequently co-occur, can mimic mood symptoms seen in BPD, make accurate diagnosis more difficult, worsen the long-term course, and compromise otherwise effective treatments.

Other comorbid conditions frequently associated with BPD include obsessive compulsive disorder, panic disorder, bulimia nervosa, impulse control disorder, ADHD, conduct disorder, and certain personality disorders.

NEUROBIOLOGY

As with many psychiatric disorders, the cause of this condition involves both *biological predisposition* and *environmental influences*. Several hypotheses have been proposed including abnormalities in:

- *Neurotransmission* (e.g., norepinephrine, serotonin)
- *Second messenger systems* (e.g., phosphoinositide cycle)
- *Biological rhythms* (e.g., sleep–wake cycle)
- *Neuroanatomy*
- *Neurophysiology* (e.g., kindling phenomenon)
- *Immune* function

From a *genetic perspective*, family studies establish a pattern of aggregation; linkage studies identify specific genomic regions associated with the disorder; and twin studies estimate concordance rates to be 14% for dizygotic twins and 57% for monozygotic twins. The absence of 100% concordance rate in monozygotic twins, however, indicates an important role for environmental factors. Therefore, a genetic–environmental interaction has been proposed in which a number of small susceptibility genes establish a gradient of liability that may trigger BPD in the context of various stressors. Of note, linkage studies report a number of genomic regions that may represent susceptibility loci for both BPD and schizophrenia. This is consistent with several clinical characteristics that these two disorders have in common.

TREATMENT OF BIPOLAR DISORDER

The optimal treatment of BPD requires early identification, medication, psychotherapy, and attention to concurrent psychiatric and medical disorders. Therefore, the management of BPD is complicated and must encompass effective treatments to minimize the frequency and severity of acute episodes, ensure long-term mood stabilization, and minimize the risk for suicide. In addition, education of patients and their families is crucial to long-term success. Although medication is clearly the necessary first step, various psychotherapeutic interventions (e.g., interpersonal social rhythm therapy [IPSRT], cognitive behavioral therapy [CBT], family focused therapy [FFT], or psychoeducation) may substantially enhance the beneficial effects of mood stabilizers.

Pharmacotherapy for Bipolar Disorder

In keeping with the multiple symptoms of BPD, several classes of psychotropics are used including:

- Mood stabilizers
- Antipsychotics
- Antidepressants
- Antianxiety/sedative-hypnotics

The *ideal mood stabilizer* should control symptoms of acute mania and depression, stabilize mood long-term, decrease suicidal propensity, minimize switches from one mood state to another, and not worsen the course of illness (e.g., induce rapid cycling). The *ideal approach* is a single-drug therapy, usually combined with psychotherapy. Table 8-1 lists the most common medications

TABLE 8-1	*Medications for Treatment of Bipolar Disorder*	
Class/Generic Name	**Trade Name (Indication)**	**Usual Daily Dosage (mg/d)**
Cation		
Lithonate, others	Lithium (A, M)	600–2,700
Antiepileptic		
Depakote	Divalproex (A)	750–2,500
Lamictal	Lamotrigine (M)	50–400
Equetro	Carbamazepine ER (A)	400–1600
Antipsychotic		
Thorazine	Chlorpromazine (A)	300–900
Zyprexa	Olanzapine (A, M, ADJ)	10–20
Risperdal	Risperidone (A, ADJ)	2–6
Seroquel	Quetiapine (A, AD, ADJ)	300–800
Abilify	Aripiprazole (A, M)	10–30
Geodon	Ziprasidone (A)	80–160
Antipsychotic plus antidepressant		
Symbyax	OLZ/FLU (AD)	6 or 12 (OLZ)
		25 or 50 (FLU)

A, acute mania; M, maintenance therapy; ADJ, adjunct; AD, acute depression;
OLZ, olanzapine; FLU, fluoxetine.
(Adapted from Janicak et al. *Principles and Practice of Psychopharmacotherapy*, 4th ed.
Philadelphia: Lippincott Williams & Wilkins; 2006.)

used to treat BPD and Table 8-2 lists their most common adverse effects.

For *bipolar mania,* if one or two adequate trials with a classic mood stabilizer (e.g., lithium *or* divalproex sodium) are insufficient, then various drug combinations are usually attempted (e.g., lithium *plus* divalproex sodium). The second-generation antipsychotics (SGAs) (e.g., olanzapine, risperidone, quetiapine, ziprasidone, and aripiprazole) have all demonstrated antimanic

| TABLE 8-2 | Common adverse effects with mood stabilizers | | | | | |

Drug	Weight Gain	Central Nervous System	EPS	Derm	QTc	HEM
Cation						
Lithium	++	+++	0	++	0	+
*a*Antiepileptic						
Divalproex DR, ER	++	++	0	+	0	+
Lamotrigine	±	+	0	+++	0	±
Carbamazepine ER	±	+++	0	+++	0	++
Antipsychotic						
Olanzapine	+++	++	+	+	0	0
Risperidone	++	+	++	+	0	0
Quetiapine	++	++	0	+	0	0
Ziprasidone	±	+	+	+	±	0
Aripiprazole	±	+	+	+	0	0
Paliperidone ER	++	+	++	+	±	0
Clozapine	+++	+	0	+	0	+++

*a*Food and Drug Administration (FDA) recently issued warning of possible increased suicidal risk with antiepileptic drugs (AEDs), particularly in patients with epilepsy.
DR, delayed release; ER, extended release; EPS, extrapyramidal side effects; QTc, corrected QT interval; Derm, dermatological; Hem, hematological; +, mild; ++, moderate; +++, substantial; 0, none; ±, Possible issue conflicting data. (Adapted from Strakowski SM, DelBello MP, Adler CM. Comparative efficacy and tolerability of drug treatments for bipolar disorder. *CNS Drugs*. 2001;15(9):701–718; Strakowski SM, DelBello MP, Adler CM, et al. Atypical antipsychotics in the treatment of bipolar disorder [Review]. *Exp Op Pharmacother*. 2003;4(5):751–760.)

properties separate from their antipsychotic effects. Therefore, they are an alternate strategy either as monotherapy or in combination with other agents.

For *bipolar depression* there is less data to guide treatment. Antidepressant monotherapy is not recommended because of the risk of further mood destabilization. The best evidence to date for less severe depressive episodes supports monotherapy with lithium, lamotrigine, or certain SGAs (quetiapine, olanzapine). Other approaches include combining mood stabilizers (e.g., lithium plus lamotrigine), a traditional mood stabilizer plus antidepressant (e.g., divalproex plus a selective serotinin reuptake inhibitor [SSRI]); or an SGA plus antidepressant (e.g., olanzapine plus fluoxetine).

Given the recurrent nature of BPD, *prevention of relapse and prophylaxis* to minimize the risk of future episodes is critical. In this context, data support the use of lithium, lamotrigine, and certain SGAs (e.g., aripiprazole, olanzapine). Other strategies include combining mood stabilizers or a mood stabilizer plus SGA.

 Ms. R was most recently treated with divalproex sodium, but it was discontinued before her second pregnancy 18 months earlier. At that time she was started on quetiapine XR 300 mg per day.

Device-Based Therapies for Bipolar Disorder

Preliminary trials indicate that device-based therapeutic alternatives for bipolar mania (e.g., delirious mania) or depression (e.g., mixed episodes) may include electroconvulsive therapy (ECT),[1,2] bright light therapy,[3] and possibly vagus nerve stimulation[4] and transcranial magnetic stimulation.[5,6]

Psychotherapy for Bipolar Disorder

Psychotherapies as adjunctive treatments to medication with the most empirical support for BPD, include:

- *Interpersonal social rhythm therapy*
- *Family focused therapy*
- *Cognitive behavioral therapy*
- *Psychoeducation*

IPSRT developed from work with interpersonal psychotherapy (IPT) for depression. The goal is to stabilize routines, increase insight into how mood is related to interpersonal issues, and help resolve interpersonal problems. Several studies report that IPSRT is an effective adjunctive treatment and delays the recurrence of mood episodes.[7]

FFT looks at family and marital relationships with the goal of improving communication and support. There are three modules: psychoeducation, communication enhancement, and problem-solving training. Several randomized controlled trials report adjunctive FFT to be effective in delaying relapse, reducing symptoms, increasing medication adherence, and improving family interactions.[8-10]

CBT focuses on challenging the thoughts and beliefs that cause long-term vulnerability to mood instability. CBT also includes components directed toward education and organization. When this approach was added to medication for relapse prevention, it improved the overall course of illness.[11] In this context, a large, multicenter study of CBT in the United Kingdom concluded that patients in the early stages of their illness or those with less frequent relapses responded better to CBT.[12] Lam et al.[11] studied CBT for relapse prevention and found significantly less episodes, shorter episodes, and fewer hospital admissions with combined treatment. When CBT was added to mood stabilizers for the treatment of the depressed phase of BPD, the time to a depressive relapse was significantly increased.[13]

Psychoeducation is conducted either in an individual or group format and focuses on developing coping skills and sharing information. Several studies report that its addition reduces symptoms and relapse rates while increasing functioning.[14-16]

CBT has also been tailored into a 10-session intervention designed to reduce suicide attempts. It has been studied in patients who recently attempted suicide and is shown to be effective in preventing suicide attempts, decreasing hopelessness, and decreasing symptoms of depression when compared to a group receiving usual care.[17,18] The use of the techniques in this protocol including problem solving, increasing social support and medication compliance may be beneficial in suicidal patients.

Combined Psychotherapy and Pharmacotherapy for Bipolar Disorder

Although pharmacotherapy is the primary intervention for BPD, the complexities of the illness and the poor outcomes with a single approach support combined interventions. Although there are several randomized, controlled trials comparing combined therapy, it is complicated to sort out which component(s) is (are) most effective. This is primarily due to the multidimensional symptoms of BPD (e.g., depression, hypomania/mania, mixed symptoms, psychosis).

In general, the combination of psychotherapy and pharmacotherapy appears to benefit by reducing symptoms, reducing relapse, increasing compliance, and improving family interactions.

Introducing Combined Treatment

Ms. R had a reduction in her symptoms after starting quetiapine XR but was experiencing significant stress at home with her two children. The dose of quetiapine XR was gradually titrated to 500 mg per day as she acclimated to its sedating effects. We then recommended that she begin FFT and IPSRT. Having been stable for many years, she initially resisted this level of care. We reinforced that she was naturally experiencing increased stress with two small children and could benefit from as much support as possible. We suggested that the treatments may not continue for long, but could improve the course of her illness. FFT focused on educating her husband about the illness because he had not seen her this symptomatic before. In addition, they worked on enhancing their communication and regulating their schedules as much as possible with two small children. IPSRT concentrated on helping her adapt to her new lifestyle and routine.

Medications are necessary to control acute exacerbations of BPD but should be combined with other approaches to improve the overall course of illness. Therefore, early introduction of various psychotherapies may further reduce symptom severity, prevent future episodes, and resolve interpersonal difficulties.

Possible discussion points include:
- *Because medication is essential for you to continue to improve, it is important that we discuss their benefits and side effects and how you can develop a strategy to stay on your medication.*
- *In addition to medication, there are other therapies that can help you stabilize your schedule and improve communication with family and friends.*
- *We would like to include your family/spouse in treatment to educate them about your illness and how they can help to improve the quality of your life.*
- *We want to help you and your family understand how this illness impacts your life.*

■ *There are several specific therapies that can help you develop new strategies to cope with your symptoms.*

In the context of BPD, the involvement of several providers is important. Therefore, open communication is a prerequisite for a successful treatment strategy.

Questions to ask the psychotherapist
■ *Which approaches are best given the patient's phase of illness and family involvement?*
■ *What specific symptoms are you targeting?*

Questions to ask the pharmacotherapist
■ *Which approaches are best given the patient's phase of illness and family involvement?*
■ *How can we insure the patient's adherence to treatment?*
■ *What side effects should we monitor, particularly as they negatively impact the patient's ability to think, function, and overall health status?*

CLINICAL RECOMMENDATIONS

Approaches to the management of BPD vary on the basis of the phase of illness including:

■ Acute *mania*
■ Acute *depression*
■ Acute *mixed symptom episode*
■ Prevention of *relapse* (i.e., maintenance)
■ Prevention of *recurrence* (i.e., prophylaxis)
■ Prevention of *suicide*

For *acute mania*, the choice of agent is dictated by such issues as severity, presence of psychotic symptoms and comorbidities (e.g., substance use disorder). With mild to moderate symptoms, mood stabilizer monotherapy (e.g., lithium, divalproex) is our recommendation. In addition, we recommend adding psychotherapy to enhance outcomes. Depending on the phase of illness, patients may benefit from psychotherapy by addressing specific symptoms, interpersonal conflicts, suicidal ideation, unstable routines, and poor insight. The choice of psychotherapy will depend on the patient's needs. With more severe symptoms, an SGA alone or combined with a classic agent are appropriate alternates. Adjunctive oral or acute injectable benzodiazepines or SGAs may help quickly reduce symptoms of agitation, insomnia, or drug withdrawal. In more severe episodes (e.g., complicated by psychosis), an SGA alone or combined with a classic mood stabilizer is recommended. With insufficient response, combining mood stabilizers can produce a more effective result. Presentations that are life threatening may require an acute trial with ECT.

For *acute depression*, lithium or quetiapine alone may suffice for milder episodes. Often, however, a combination of medications may be required, including:

■ Mood stabilizer plus antidepressant
■ Olanzapine plus fluoxetine (olanzapine–fluoxetine combination [OFC])
■ Quetiapine plus classic mood stabilizer
■ ECT may be a life-saving option (e.g., highly suicidal, manic delirium)

Once an acute episode has improved, the focus then turns to the more difficult task of *relapse and recurrence prevention*. Frequently, a "top down, bottom up" strategy is needed. This entails the use of an agent more effective in delaying manic symptoms (e.g., lithium) combined with an agent more effective in developing depressive symptoms (e.g., lamotrigine). It is at this stage that adjunctive psychotherapy also plays a critical role.

In the latter context, BPD receives a lot of attention in self-help books and from personal accounts. Miklowitz, who developed FFT, provides useful information in *"The Bipolar Survival Guide."*[19] In addition, Jones et al.[20] wrote a very useful self-help guide. Clinicians less familiar with these interventions for BPD may find Barlow's[21] comprehensive textbook instructive. Basco and Rush[22] and Newman et al.[23] also outline treatment with CBT in their textbooks. Finally, Frank[24] developed a clinician's guide to IPSRT.

Ms. R's bipolar illness had been stable for many years, so she was naturally overwhelmed and frightened at the reoccurrence. Significant time was spent with her husband, helping him understand BPD, and to accept this aspect of his wife. In addition, adaptation to their more stressful life situation will require significant time and effort.

Figures 8-1, 8-2, and 8-3 outline the approach we recommend.

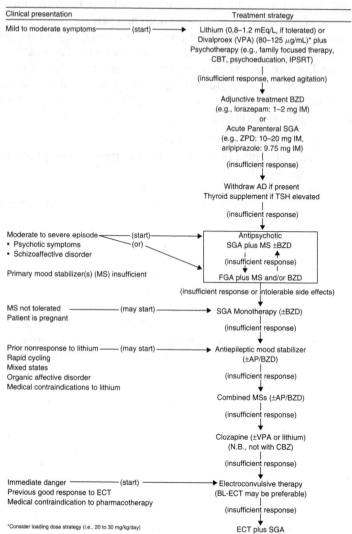

FIGURE 8-1 ■ Treatment of acute mania. CBT, cognitive behavioral therapy; IPSRT, interpersonal social rhythm therapy; BZD, benzodiazepine; SGA, second-generation antipsychotic; ZPD, ziprasidone; AD, antidepressant; TSH, thyroid-stimulating hormone; FGA, first-generation antipsychotic; AP, antipsychotic; CBZ, carbamazepine; BL, bilateral; ECT, electroconvulsive therapy. (Adapted from Janicak PG, Davis JM, Preskorn SH, et al. *Principles and Practice of Psychopharmacotherapy*, 4th ed. Philadelphia: Lippincott Williams & Wilkins; 2006.)

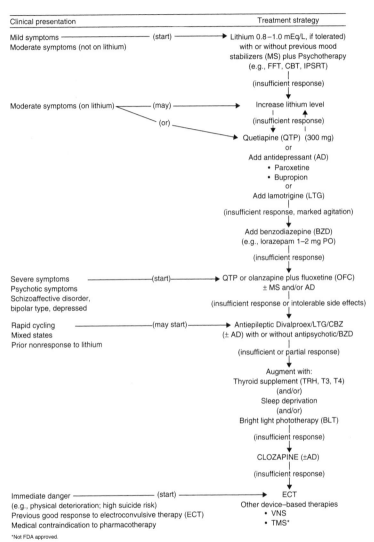

FIGURE 8-2 ■ Treatment of acute bipolar depression. FFT, family focused therapy; CBT, cognitive behavioral therapy; IPSRT, interpersonal social rhythm therapy; CBZ, carbamazepine; TRH, thyrotroph releasing hormone; VNS, vagus nerve stimulation; TMS, transcranial magnetic stimulation. (Adapted from Janicak PG, Davis JM, Preskorn SH, et al. *Principles and Practice of Psychopharmacotherapy*, 4th ed. Philadelphia: Lippincott Williams & Wilkins; 2006.)

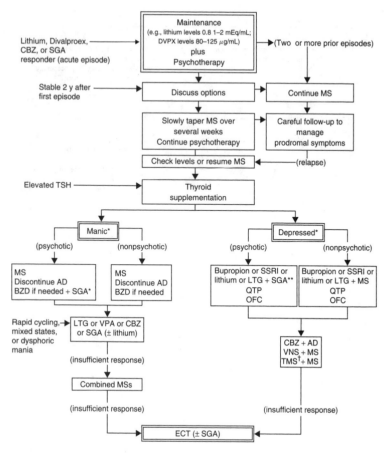

*Psychotherapy should be continued.
**Consider RISP microspheres in noncompliant patients or with poor oral absorption or rapid metabolism.
†Not FDA approved.

FIGURE 8-3 ■ Maintenance strategy for bipolar disorder. CBZ, carbamazepine; SGA, second-generation antipsychotic; DVPX, divalproex; MS, mood stabilizer; TSH, thyroid-stimulating hormone; AD, antidepressant; BZD, benzodiazepine; SSRI, selective serotonin reuptake inhibitor; LTG, lamotrigine; QTP, quetiapine; OFC, olanzapine plus fluoxetine; VNS, vagus nerve stimulation; TMS, transcranial magnetic stimulation; ECT, electroconvulsive therapy; RISP, risperidone; FDA, U.S. Food and Drug Administration. (Adapted from Janicak PG, Davis JM, Preskorn SH, et al. *Principles and Practice of Psychopharmacotherapy*, 4th ed. Philadelphia: Lippincott Williams & Wilkins; 2006.)

Learning points

- Diagnosing and treating BPD presents a considerable challenge to clinicians.
- Various classes of mood stabilizers are effective when used alone or in combination.
- Psychotherapy plays an important adjunctive role, particularly during the maintenance and prophylactic phases of treatment.

REFERENCES

1. Karmacharya R, England ML, Ongur D. Delirious mania: Clinical features and treatment response. *J Affect Disord.* 2008; Epub ahead of print.
2. Valenti M, Benabarre A, Garcia-Amador M, et al. Electroconvulsive therapy in the treatment of mixed states in bipolar disorder. *Eur Psychiatry.* 2008;23(1):53–56.
3. Sit D, Wisner KL, Hanusa BH, et al. Light therapy for bipolar disorder: A case series in women. *Bipolar Disord.* 2007;9(8):918–927.
4. Marangell LB, Suppes T, Zboyan HA, et al. A 1-year pilot study of vagus nerve stimulation in treatment-resistant rapid-cycling bipolar disorder. *J Clin Psychiatry.* 2008:e1–e7; Epub ahead of print.
5. Li X, Nahas Z, Anderson B, et al. Can left prefrontal rTMS be used as a maintenance treatment for bipolar depression. *Depress Anxiety.* 2004;20(2):98–100.
6. Michael N, Erfurth A. Treatment of bipolar mania with right prefrontal rapid transcranial magnetic stimulation. *J Affect Disord.* 2004; 78(3):253–257.
7. Frank E, Kupfer DJ, Thase ME, et al. Two year outcomes for interpersonal social rhythm therapy in individuals with bipolar disorder. *Arch Gen Psychiatry.* 2005;62(9):996–1004.
8. Miklowitz DJ, Otto MW, Frank E, et al. Psychosocial treatments from bipolar depression: A 1 year randomized trial from the systematic treatment enhancement program. *Arch Gen Psychiatry.* 2007;64(4): 419–427.
9. Simoneau TL, Miklowitz DJ, Richards JA, et al. Bipolar disorder and family communication: Effects of a psychoeducational treatment program. *J Abnorm Psychol.* 1999;108:588–597.
10. Rea MM, Tompson MC, Miklowitz DJ, et al. Family-focused treatment versus individual treatment for bipolar disorder: Results of a randomized clinical trial. *J Consult Clin Psychol.* 2003;71(3):482–492.

11. Lam DH, Watkins ER, Hayward P, et al. A randomized controlled study of cognitive therapy for relapse prevention for bipolar disorder: Outcome of the first year. *Arch Gen Psychiatry*. 2003;60(2): 145–152.

12. Scott J, Paykel E, Morriss R, et al. Cognitive behaviour therapy for severe and recurrent bipolar disorders: A randomized controlled trial. *Br J Psychiatry*. 2006;188:313–320.

13. Ball JR, Mitchell PB, Corry JC, et al. A randomized controlled trial of cognitive therapy for bipolar disorder: Focus on long-term change. *J Clin Psychiatry*. 2006;67(2):277–286.

14. Perry A, Tarrier N, Morriss R, et al. Randomized controlled trial of efficacy of teaching patient with bipolar disorder. *Br Med J*. 1999;318(7177):149–153.

15. Colom F, Vieta E, Martinez-Aran A, et al. A randomized trial on the efficacy of group psychoeducation in the prophylaxis of recurrences in bipolar patients whose disease is in remission. *Arch Gen Psychiatry*. 2003;60(4):402–407.

16. Simon GE, Ludman EJ, Unützer J, et al. Randomized trial of population-based care program for people with bipolar disorder. *Psychol Med*. 2005;35(1):13–24.

17. Tarrier N, Taylor R, Gooding P. Cognitive behavioral interventions to reduce suicide behavior: A systematic review and meta-analysis. *Behav. Modif.* 2008;32(1):77–108.

18. Brown GK, Have TT, Henriques GR, et al. Cognitive therapy for the prevention of suicide attempts a randomized controlled trial. *JAMA*. 294(5):563–570.

19. Miklowitz DJ. *The bipolar disorder survival guide*. New York: The Guilford Press; 2002.

20. Jones S, Hayward P, Lam D. *Coping with bipolar disorder: a guide to living with manic depression*. Oxford, England: Oneworld Publications; 2002.

21. Barlow DH, ed. *Clinical handbook of psychological disorders*, 4th ed. New York: The Guilford Press; 2007:421–462.

22. Basco MR, Rush AJ. *Cognitive behavioral therapy for bipolar disorder*, 2nd ed. New York: The Guilford Press; 2005.

23. Newman CV, Leahy RL, Beck AT, et al. *Bipolar disorder: a cognitive therapy approach*. Washington, DC: American Psychological Association; 2001.

24. Frank E. *Treating bipolar disorder: a clinician's guide to interpersonal and social rhythm therapy*. New York: The Guilford Press; 2005.

SUGGESTED READINGS

Fisher JR, O'Donohue WT, eds. *Practitioner's guide to evidence-based psychotherapy*. New York, NY: Springer; 2006.

Janicak PG. Bipolar disorder. In: Albrecht GL, ed. *The encyclopedia of disability*, 5 Vols. Thousand Oaks: Sage Publications; 2006:175–176.

Janicak PG, Davis JM, Preskorn SH, et al. *Principles and practice of psychopharmacotherapy*, 4th ed. Philadelphia: Lippincott Williams & Wilkins; 2006.

Strakowski SM, DelBello MP, Adler CM. Comparative efficacy and tolerability of drug treatments for bipolar disorder. *CNS Drugs*. 2001; 15(9):701–718.

Strakowski SM, DelBello MP, Adler CM, et al. Atypical antipsychotics in the treatment of bipolar disorder (Review). *Exp Op Pharmacother*. 2003;4(5):751–760.

Borderline Personality

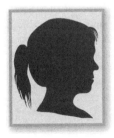

Ms. S

Ms. S is a 23-year-old, single woman who was seen in the emergency department following a suicide attempt and admitted to the hospital for further assessment. She reported feeling out of control and overwhelmed following the break up of a 6-month relationship. As a result, she took an overdose of acetaminophen and called her family soon after. She had been in and out of treatment for the previous 4 years but had not seen her therapist in the last 7 months.

Borderline personality disorder is listed as a Cluster B subtype which includes antisocial, histrionic, and narcissistic personality disorders as well. It is characterized by:

- Unstable *affect*
- Stormy interpersonal *relationships*
- Behavioral *dyscontrol*

The estimated prevalence of this Axis II disorder is 1% to 2%. It is often complicated by Axis I mood disorders (e.g., 25% to 75% experience major depression, 5% to 20% meet criteria for bipolar disorder). In addition, 70% abuse alcohol or other drugs and 25% of bulimic patients also meet criteria for this personality disorder. Self-destructive and suicidal behaviors are common. Physical or sexual abuse, trauma, and neglect are frequent antecedents to this condition. Physical disorders of the central nervous system (CNS) (e.g., neurodevelopmental, acquired brain insults) have also been considered as potential predisposing factors.

DIFFERENTIAL DIAGNOSIS

Affective, impulsive, and psychotic symptoms frequently complicate this condition. These presentations are the basis for the major differential diagnostic considerations, including:

- Mood disorders
- Impulse control disorders
- Schizophrenia

Ms. S has a long history of interpersonal conflicts, impulsivity, outbursts of anger, and repeated suicide attempts. She describes a labile mood and easily becomes upset. She was diagnosed with bipolar disorder in the past but currently only meets criteria for borderline personality disorder due to the absence of a primary mood component.

NEUROBIOLOGY

The frequent observation that family members of borderline patients often manifest impulse control disorders suggests a possible *genetic-related condition*. Disinhibition is a hallmark of such disorders and may contribute to the parental abuse patterns that pervade the history of borderline patients.

Another line of evidence is the observation that *injuries to the prefrontal and orbitofrontal cortical areas* can produce borderline-like behaviors. Further, both structural and functional neuroimaging studies also support dysfunction in the frontolimbic network.[1]

TREATMENT OF BORDERLINE PERSONALITY DISORDER

Pharmacotherapy of Borderline Personality Disorder

It is difficult to do well-controlled clinical trials with highly disturbed, suicidal patients such as those with severe borderline features. Therefore, most studies involve small sample sizes. The three leading major medication strategies include the use of antidepressants (ADs), antiepileptic drugs (AEDs), and second-generation antipsychotics (SGAs). While benzodiazepines are also frequently prescribed; problems with abuse, dependency, and possible further disinhibition should limit their use (see Table 9-1).

Antidepressants. Two small-sample, controlled studies provided some evidence that monoamine oxidase inhibitors (MAOIs) such as tranyclypromine may benefit borderline personality and related disorders. Whereas open trials with selective serotonin reuptake inhibitors (SSRIs) (e.g., fluoxetine and sertraline) indicated these agents may be most effective for impulsive aggression and irritability; placebo-controlled trials supported their benefit for affective instability and anger but not for impulsivity, aggression, unstable relationships, suicidality, and global functioning.[2,3]

TABLE 9-1	Medications for Treatment of Borderline Personality Disorder	
Class/Generic Name	**Common Trade Name**	**Daily Dose Range (mg)**
Antidepressants		
SSRIs (e.g., fluoxetine)	Prozac	10–40
Antiepileptics		
Lamotrigine	Lamictal	50–200
Topiramate	Topamax	25–200
Divalproex	Depakote	250–2,000
Second-Generation Antipsychotics		
Aripiprazole	Abilify	2–15
Olanzapine	Zyprexa	2.5–7.5
Quetiapine	Seroquel	200–800

While both MAOI and SSRI trials found these agents helpful for impulsivity, some also demonstrated effectiveness in controlling mood. As the SSRIs produce AD as well as anti-impulsivity and antiaggression properties, they are frequently used in this population. Because these patients are prone to suicide attempts, it is important to remember that first-generation ADs (e.g., tricyclic antidepressants [TCAs], MAOIs) are potentially lethal in overdose. By contrast, the SSRIs are very safe.

Antiepileptic Drugs. Open and randomized controlled trials indicate that AEDs (e.g., lamotrigine, topiramate, divalproex) may be more effective than ADs in controlling various symptoms of borderline personality disorder.

In an open case series, Pinto and Akiskal[4] found that several treatment-resistant borderline patients (particularly those with a bipolar component to their illness) had a robust response to lamotrigine over a 1-year period. In addition, one patient had an excellent response to divalproex. More recent, controlled trials support the benefit of lamotrigine for both short-term and long-term control of aggression and anger in women.[5,6] Data also support the benefit of topiramate to manage anger, aggression, and depressive symptoms in both women and men.[7,8]

Antipsychotics. Borderline patients often present with psychotic features. In this context, several placebo-controlled studies indicate that antipsychotics are efficacious in these patients. More recently, trials with aripiprazole demonstrated both acute and longer-term benefit over 18 months.[9,10] Further, this drug positively impacted most symptoms (i.e., not just psychosis) associated with borderline personality disorder. An observational trial of acute parenteral olanzapine also demonstrated good tolerability and efficacy for agitated borderline patients.

In summary, the evidence indicates that AEDs and SGAs may supplant ADs as the preferred medication strategy.[11] In addition, the specific medication choice should be dictated by symptom presentation and safety/tolerability profile. In this context, polypharmacy is discouraged and usually unnecessary.[12] Of note, the U.S. Food and Drug Administration (FDA) has recently issued a warning regarding a possible increased risk of suicidal behavior with various AEDs.

Psychotherapy for Borderline Personality Disorder

Currently, there are two empirically supported treatments for borderline personality disorder: dialectic behavioral therapy (DBT) and mentalization based treatment (MBT). Both have been assessed in randomized controlled trials and found efficacious.

DBT was developed as an outpatient treatment by Linehan[13] based on cognitive behavioral principles. It emphasizes a biological predisposition to emotional dysregulation combined with an environment that invalidates the patient's experiences. This interaction is very complicated with each component impacting the other (i.e., the emotional dysregulation leads to invalidation and vice versa). Treatment focuses on learning to regulate emotions, increasing interpersonal effectiveness, tolerating distress, and increasing mindfulness. *Mindfulness* is a key component of DBT and includes skills in observing, describing, and participating effectively in a nonjudgmental, organized manner. Important tenets are balancing change and acceptance. Several controlled trials reported that DBT decreased parasuicidal behavior (e.g., suicidal threats, self-injurious behavior), lowered the frequency and length of inpatient hospitalizations, decreased treatment dropouts and increased skill areas (e.g., tolerating distress, regulating emotions, mindfulness).

Mentalization based treatment (MBT) is based on attachment theory and was developed as a partial hospitalization program by Bateman and Fonagy.[14] It focuses on relationship patterns and the nonconscious factors that interfere with making change. Mentalization describes the ability to interpret the actions of other people. This is particularly difficult for individuals with borderline personality disorder. In randomized controlled trials, MBT was effective in reducing suicidal behavior, the number of inpatient hospitalizations, and symptoms of anxiety and depression.[15]

Combined Psychotherapy and Pharmacotherapy for Borderline Personality Disorder

Borderline personality disorder presents with a multitude of symptoms, making it difficult to develop a simple pharmacologic strategy. Hence, establishing the benefits of combined psychotherapy and pharmacotherapy is even more complicated. In this context, Soler et al.[16] randomized 60 patients with borderline personality disorder to DBT plus olanzapine or DBT plus placebo. Subjects in the DBT plus olanzapine group evidenced lower scores on measures of depression and anxiety. In addition, compared with the placebo group the combined treatment approach decreased impulsive/aggressive behaviors. The DBT plus olanzapine group, however, gained significantly more weight and experienced a significant increase in cholesterol levels.

Owing to the high incidence of suicidal and parasuicidal symptoms in borderline personality disorder, communication is very important if combined treatment is conducted by separate treaters. Risk management is also a major concern of clinicians treating this disorder. As a result, treatment planning, crisis intervention, and communication between clinicians should occur frequently and be carefully documented. In addition, clinicians must collaborate to maintain a consistent message and intervention to the patient.

Questions to ask the psychotherapist
- *What symptoms are you targeting?*
- *What approach or approaches are you considering?*
- *How frequently should we communicate regarding our patient?*
- *Can the patient reach you quickly during a crisis?*

Questions to ask the pharmacotherapist
- *What symptoms are you targeting?*

- *Are you planning any medication adjustments?*
- *What would be the best way for us to communicate?*
- *In addition to our regular contact, what symptom changes would you like to be contacted for?*
- *How are you advising the patient to use their medications so I can reinforce your treatment?*
- *How would you like to handle our patient's thoughts of suicide?*
- *What are your criteria for hospitalizing our patient?*

Ms. S, following admission and a brief assessment, was discharged to a day hospital program specializing in DBT. She had previously been in numerous similar programs and was initially resistant. With support and encouragement from staff, however, she agreed to attend the initial evaluation. The program provided a very structured approach including group and individual therapy, as well as telephone consultation. In addition, her psychiatrist prescribed lamotrigine (25 mg per day with gradual titration to 200 mg per day as tolerated over several weeks) to address both her impulsivity and possible bipolar disorder. MS. S also began the initial stages of DBT which focused on orienting her to treatment and establishing a commitment to work together.

CLINICAL RECOMMENDATIONS

We recommend combined treatment with the primary therapeutic approach being DBT or MBT plus symptom-specific pharmacologic interventions. Therefore, significant depression and suicidality would suggest an SSRI. Impulsive aggression may benefit more from an AED such as lamotrigine or topiramate. With psychotic symptoms and aggression, an SGA is a reasonable option. Given the metabolic issues with olanzapine, we would consider a trial with aripiprazole first.

Owing to the severity of borderline personality disorder alternate strategies for treatment are relatively limited. Although there are several popular self-help books, none have been validated. Linehan,[13] the developer of DBT for borderline personality disorder, published a skills training manual. Linehan has also published several DBT manuals for clinicians.[13,17] The most recent focuses on the use of DBT across several disorders and settings (e.g., substance dependence, eating disorders, inpatients, outpatients, families, adolescents). Several books focus on coping with borderline personality disorder.[18,19] Other sources for clinicians who are unfamiliar with the recommended psychotherapeutic interventions include Barlow's chapter on DBT and a review of MBT.[20]

Ms. S began the process of committing to treatment. This helped reduce her suicidal and negative behaviors, providing the opportunity to acquire new behavioral/coping skills. Because medication was very important to the patient, she continued treatment with lamotrigine (200 mg/day), as well.

Figure 9-1 outlines the strategy we would recommend for treatment of borderline personality disorder.

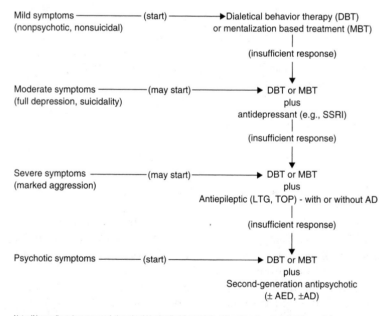

Note: If benzodiazepines are used, they should be for disabling anxiety, at low doses for only a short time period.

FIGURE 9-1 ■ Treatment strategy for borderline personality disorder. SSRI, selective serotonin reuptake inhibitor; LTG, lamotrigine; AD, antidepressant; AED, antiepileptic drug.

Learning points

- DBT and MBT are effective psychotherapies and the primary treatment approach for borderline personality disorder.
- Pharmacotherapy is a useful adjunct treatment to manage specific symptoms (e.g., mood instability, impulsivity, psychosis) associated with borderline personality disorder.
- Limited trial data and extensive clinical experience indicate that combining psychotherapy with symptom-specific medication therapy may provide a more robust benefit.

REFERENCES

1. Schmahl C, Bremner JD. Neuroimaging in borderline personality disorder. *J Psychiatr Res*. 2006;40(5):419–427.
2. Nose M, Cipriani A, Biancosino B, et al. Efficacy of pharmacology against core traits of borderline personality disorder: Meta-analysis of randomized controlled trials. *Int Clin Psychopharmacol*. 2006;21(6): 345–353.
3. Binks CA, Fenton M, McCarthy L, et al. Pharmacological interventions for people with borderline personality disorder. *Cochrane Database Syst Rev*. 2006;1:CD005653.
4. Pinto OC, Akiskal HS. Lamotrigine as a promising approach to borderline personality: An open case series without concurrent DSM-IV major mood disorder. *J Affect Disord*. 1998;51:333–343.
5. Tritt K, Nickel C, Lahmann C, et al. Lamotrigine treatment of aggression in female borderline-patients: A randomized, double-blind, placebo-controlled study. *J Psychopharmacol*. 2005;19(3):287–291.
6. Leiberich PK, Nickel MK, Tritt K, et al. Lamotrigine treatment of aggression in female borderline patients, part II: An 18-month follow-up. *J Psychopharmacol*. 2008;28; Epub ahead of print.
7. Nickel MK, Nickel C, mitterlehner FO, et al. Topiramate treatment of aggression in female borderline personality disorder patients: A double-bline, placebo-controlled study. *J Clin Psychiatry*. 2004; 65(11):1515–1519.
8. Nickel MK, Nickel C, Kaplan P, et al. Treatment of aggression with topiramate in male borderline patients: A double-blind, placebo-controlled study. *Biol Psychiatry*. 2005;57(5):495–499.

9. Nickel MK, Muehlbacher M, Nickel C, et al. Aripiprazole in the treatment of patients with borderline personality disorder: A double-blind, placebo-controlled study. *Am J Psychiatry*. 2006;163(5): 833–838.
10. Nickel MK, Loew TH, Pedrosa Gil F. Aripiprazole in treatment of borderline patients, part II: An 18-month follow-up. *Psychopharmacology*. 2007;191(4):1023–1026.
11. Abraham PF, Calabrese JR. Evidence-based pharmacologic treatment of borderline personality disorder: A shift from SSRIs to anticonvulsants and atypical antipsychotics? *J Affect Disord*. 2008;(25), Epub ahead of print.
12. Zanarini MC. Update on pharmacotherapy of borderline personality disorder. *Curr Psychiatry Res*. 2004;6(1):66–70.
13. Linehan MM. *Cognitive behavioral therapy for borderline personality disorder*. New York: The Guilford Press; 1993.
14. Batemen A, Fonagy P. Treatment of borderline personality disorder with psychoanalytically oriented partial hospitalization: An 18 month follow up. *Am J Psychiatry*. 2001;158:36–42.
15. Batemann A, Fonagy P. 8 year follow up of patients treated for borderline personality disorder. Mentalization based treatment versus treatment as usual. *AM J Psychiatry*. 2008;165(5):631–638.
16. Soler J, Pascual JC, Campins J, et al. Double-blind, placebo controlled study of dialectical behavior therapy plus olanzapine for borderline personality disorder. *Am J Psychiatry*. 2005;162(6):1221–1224.
17. Linehan MM, Dimeff LA, Koerner K. *Dialectical behavior therapy in clinical practice: applications across disorders and settings*. New York: The Guilford Press; 2007.
18. Bockian NR, Villagran NE, Porr V. *New hope for people with borderline personality disorder: your friendly, authoritative guide to the latest in traditional and complementary solutions*. New York: Random House; 2002.
19. Thorton MF. *Eclipses: behind the borderline personality disorder*. Monte Sano Publishing; 1997.
20. Barlow DH. *Clinical handbook of psychological disorders*. New York: The Guilford Press; 2007:365–420.

SUGGESTED READINGS

Batemen A, Fonagy P. Treatment of borderline personality disorder with psychoanalytically oriented partial hospitalization: An 18 month follow up. *Am J Psychiatry*. 2001;158:36–42.
Binks CA, Fenton M, McCarthy L. Pharmacological interventions for people with borderline personality disorder. *Cochrane Database Syst Rev*. 2006;1:CD005653.

Fisher JR, O'Donohue WT, eds. *Practitioner's guide to evidence-based psychotherapy*. New York, NY: Springer; 2006.

Linehan MM. *Skills training manual for treating borderline personality disorder*. New York: The Guilford Press; 1993.

Loew TH, Nickel MK, Muehlbacher M, et al. Topiramate treatment for women with borderline personality disorder: A double-blind, placebo-controlled study. *J Clin Psycopharmacol*. 2006;26(1): 61–66.

Soler J, Pascual JC, Campins J, et al. Double-blind, placebo controlled study of dialectical behavior therapy plus olanzapine for borderline personality disorder. *Am J Psychiatry*. 2007;162(6);1221–1224.

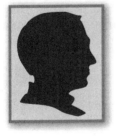

10

Generalized Anxiety Disorder

LEARNING OBJECTIVES

1. Understand the differences and relationship between pharmacotherapy and psychotherapy for the treatment of generalized anxiety disorder.
2. Develop strategies for combined or sequenced treatment approaches for generalized anxiety disorder.
3. Enhance skills to negotiate these treatment approaches with patients.

Mr. X

Mr. X is a 60-year-old, married man referred by his primary care physician (PCP). He has experienced a very difficult year with the loss of his job and his wife's diagnosis of breast cancer. He describes feeling worried and anxious on most days for several months. He also reports feeling on edge and "physically tense." His dentist has also noted that he is grinding his teeth at night. He describes himself as a worrier but recently it has become uncontrollable, even disrupting his sleep. His PCP has medically cleared him.

Stress, anxiety, and worry are normal experiences that incorporate qualities of fear and related emotions. Such feelings can ensure adaptation and survival, but when excessive, may impair one's ability to function. The Diagnostic and Statistical Manual of Mental Disorders (DSM-IV-TR) defines generalized anxiety disorder (GAD) as excessive anxiety or worry occurring more days than not for at least 6 months about a number of events or activities (e.g., work or school performance). In addition, the individual finds it difficult to control the worry. Three or more of the following symptoms should be present:

- *Restlessness*
- *Fatigue*
- Poor *concentration*
- *Irritability*
- Muscle *tension*
- Disturbed *sleep*

Approximately 50% of patients with a complaint of anxiety will meet criteria for GAD. Related symptoms increase overall medical expenses including unnecessary consultations. Further, antianxiety agents are the fourth most prescribed medications in all of medicine. Available evidence indicates that GAD may last for many years with waxing and waning symptoms, often complicated by other intercurrent physical or psychiatric disorders. Although a DSM-IV-TR–derived diagnosis requires a duration of at least 6 months, clinicians often encounter very symptomatic patients who do not meet this specific duration criterion. Therefore, in addition to formalized diagnostic criteria, clinical judgment and experience are critical in deciding when anxiety is a discrete disorder requiring primary treatment and when it is a manifestation of another disorder.

Mr. X describes feeling very fatigued; having trouble concentrating; and worrying about his wife, children, house, and work. Owing to his worry, he works longer hours, calls his children daily to check on them, and has started several home repair projects to cope. He denies other mood symptoms. Approximately 20 years ago his PCP recommended a selective serotonin reuptake inhibitor (SSRI) to better manage feeling anxious and overwhelmed. The patient could not recall the name of the medication, took it only briefly, and reports that it did not help.

DIFFERENTIAL DIAGNOSIS

Differential psychiatric diagnostic considerations include:

- *Substance-induced* disorders (e.g., caffeine intoxication)
- *Adjustment* disorder with anxious mood (characterized by lack of full symptom criteria for GAD and the presence of a recognized psychosocial stressor)
- *Psychotic, eating* or *mood* disorders in which anxiety is related to the underlying condition

In addition, numerous *medical disorders* (e.g., hyperthyroidism, cardiovascular disease) may be complicated by anxious features.

NEUROBIOLOGY OF GENERALIZED ANXIETY DISORDER

Several *neurotransmitters, neuropeptides, neurohormones,* and *cellular mediators* are implicated in the pathophysiology of anxiety disorders. In this context, agents that are effective for treating GAD include those working through:

- *Gamma-aminobutyric acid (GABA)* system
- *Serotonin* system
- *Noradrenergic* system

In addition, *behavioral models* are critical in understanding anxiety disorders and their therapeutic modulation. For example, conflict procedures (i.e., subjects experience the opposing impulses of desire and fear) have helped to conceptualize these conditions and are the basis for certain psychotherapeutic strategies.

TREATMENT OF GENERALIZED ANXIETY DISORDER

Pharmacotherapy for Generalized Anxiety Disorder

Several psychotropics and antiepileptic drugs have demonstrated efficacy for GAD. Table 10-1 lists these agents and their usual daily dosing ranges.

TABLE 10-1	Medications for Treatment of Generalized Anxiety Disorder	

Class/Generic Name	Common Trade Name	Daily Dose Range (mg/d)
Benzodiazepines		
Chlordiazepoxide	Librium, others	10–100
Diazepam	Valium, others	2–40
Oxazepam	Serax, others	30–120
Chlorazepate	Tranxene, others	15–60
Lorazepam	Ativan	1–10
Prazepam	Centrax	20–60
Halazepam	Paxipam	60–160
Alprazolam	Xanax	0.75–4
Serotonergic agents		
SSRIs	Sertraline, others	25–250
Buspirone	BuSpar	15–60
Trazodone[a]	Desyrel	50–100
Noradrenergic agents		
Propranolol[a]	Inderal	30–120
Clonidine[a]	Catapres	0.1–0.5
Serotonergic/noradrenergic agents		
Venlafaxine XR	Effexor XR	75–375
Duloxetine[a]	Cymbalta	20–60
Antihistamines		
Diphenhydramine[a]	Benadryl	25–50
Hydroxyzine[b]	Atarax	25–50
Antiepileptic drugs		
Gabapentin[a]	Neurontin	300–5,000
Pregabalin[c]	Lyrica	150–600

Class/Generic Name	Common Trade Name	Daily Dose Range (mg/d)
TABLE 10-1 *Medications for Treatment of Generalized Anxiety Disorder (continued)*		
Tiagabine[a]	Gabitril	4–16
Divalproex[a]	Depakote, others	250–2,000
Natural remedies		
Kava	Kavatrol	210–240 mg/kL

[a]Not approved by the U.S. Food and Drug Administration (FDA) for anxiety or sleep disorders.
[b]Symptomatic relief of anxiety and tension associated with psychoneurosis and as an adjunct in organic disease states in which anxiety is manifest.
[c]Studies in social phobia, GAD; no FDA approval yet.
BZD, benzodiazepine; CRF, corticotropin-releasing factor; NMDA, N-methyl-D-aspartate; GAD, general anxiety disorder.
(Adapted from Janicak PG, Davis JM, Preskorn SH, et al. *Principles and Practice of Psychopharmacotherapy*, 4th ed. Philadelphia: Lippincott Williams & Wilkins; 2006.)

Benzodiazepines. Although other drugs exert anxiolytic effects, the benzodiazepines (BZDs) are still commonly used to treat GAD. A meta-analysis of well-controlled studies found these agents superior to placebo and comparable to each other in the short-term management of GAD.[1] Almost all studies indicated that BZDs quickly reduce symptoms in many patients, with most improvement occurring during the first week. Patients most likely to respond demonstrate:

- *Acute, severe* anxiety
- Precipitating *stressors*
- *Low level of depression* or *interpersonal* problems
- *No previous treatment*, or a *good response* to earlier treatment
- Expectation of *recovery*
- Desire to use *medication*
- Awareness that symptoms are *psychological*
- Some improvement in the *first week of treatment*

Many derive sustained benefit from only short-term use of a BZD. Therefore, treatment should be with the lowest possible dose for the shortest possible time. In more chronic courses, doses should be flexible rather than arbitrarily fixed and taken intermittently at a time of increased symptoms rather than on a daily schedule. In general, 1 to 7 days of treatment are recommended for reaction to an acute situational stress, although 1 to 6 weeks of treatment may be needed for short-term anxiety due to specific life events.

Because disorders such as GAD are often chronic, long-term treatment may be required. However, even when long-term BZD therapy is appropriate, periodic reassessment of efficacy, safety, and necessity is appropriate given problems associated with these agents such as:

- Excessive daytime *drowsiness*
- *Cognitive impairment* and *confusion*
- *Psychomotor impairment* and a risk of *falls*
- *Intoxication,* even on therapeutic dosages
- *Respiratory* problems
- *Abuse* and *dependence*

Therefore, clinical judgment plays a major role in the decision to continue BZD anxiolytic treatment beyond 4 to 6 weeks. To lessen the likelihood of adverse effects and withdrawal phenomena, many experts recommend limiting BZD use to 4 months or less and to gradually taper patients off these agents as tolerated.

The chronic nature of anxiety disorders and the frequency of eventual relapse after treatment discontinuation, however, suggest that in some patients long-term treatment is indicated. Unfortunately, only limited controlled data exist on the efficacy of chronic administration. In this context, strategies to avoid dependence or withdrawal symptoms include:

- Regular *monitoring*
- The *lowest possible doses* to achieve the therapeutic effect
- *Intermittent and flexible dosing schedules*
- *Gradual dose reduction*

Antidepressants. These agents are increasingly considered as first-line treatment for GAD because they:

- Are *as effective as BZDs* in controlled trials.
- Can *alleviate both anxiety and depression*, which commonly co-occur.

■ Pose *minimal risks for dependence and withdrawal* symptoms compared to BZDs, particularly with long-term treatment.

■ Have a *different adverse effect profile* than BZDs, which may be more tolerable for certain patients.

Selective Serotonin Reuptake Inhibitors. Paroxetine has demonstrated an excellent efficacy and safety/tolerability profile in placebo-controlled trials for both the short- and long-term treatment of GAD.[2,3] Sertraline and escitalopram have also demonstrated comparable efficacy to paroxetine. Initial worsening of anxiety, gastrointestinal symptoms, and sexual dysfunction are the most frequent adverse effects experienced with the SSRIs.

Tricyclics. Although some first-generation antidepressants (e.g., imipramine, amitriptyline) have also demonstrated anxiolytic properties, adverse effect profiles limit their utilizability (see Table 2-5).

Dual Serotonergic/Noradrenergic Agents. Venlafaxine extended-release formulation (XR) was efficacious for GAD without associated major depression in several acute, outpatient clinical trials.[4] Further, a 6-month, randomized, placebo-controlled maintenance trial found this agent safe and effective in patients with GAD.[5] At the conclusion of this study, 67% of the patients on venlafaxine XR (75–225 mg per day) versus only 33% of the patients on placebo were rated much or very much improved. Nausea, somnolence, and dry mouth are common, patient-reported adverse events with venlafaxine XR.

Buspirone. This azapirone anxiolytic acts as a 5-HT_{1A} agonist. A major advantage is the lack of BZD-type adverse effects, abuse potential, or withdrawal syndrome. Potential disadvantages are the multiple daily dosing regimen, a slower onset of action than the BZDs, ineffectiveness for panic symptoms, and lack of cross tolerance with BZDs (i.e., will not block withdrawal symptoms when switching from a BZD). Generally, this agent is well tolerated with the most common adverse effects being gastrointestinal symptoms, headache, and initial restlessness.

Antiepileptic Drugs. Agents such as gabapentin, tiagabine, and Divalproex have all shown preliminary benefit for GAD. The best studied antiepileptic drug (AED), pregabalin, has been approved for treatment of GAD in other countries. It appears to produce rapid and comparable anxiolytic effects to BZDs without many of their drawbacks. Adverse effects vary by specific AED agent but are generally mild in nature with most patients demonstrating eventual acclimation and low (usually placebo level) dropout rates in the clinical trials. Of note, the FDA has recently issued a warning about possible increased suicidality with various AEDs.

Other Agents. Other agents considered for treatment of GAD include:

- Antihistamines (e.g., hydroxyzine)
- Second-generation antipsychotics (SGAs) (e.g., quetiapine)
- Natural remedies (e.g., Kava)

Although there is data from controlled trials for some of these agents, none have FDA approval and some may carry significant risks (e.g., hepatotoxicity with Kava).

Psychotherapy for Generalized Anxiety Disorder

The most validated psychotherapy for GAD is cognitive behavioral therapy (CBT). It was found more effective than supportive therapy, psychodynamic therapy, and no therapy (e.g., wait list controls).[6,7] Determining which component or combination of components is most efficacious, however, is difficult. Several meta-analyses of CBT compared with relaxation training report mixed results either demonstrating that CBT alone was equivalent to relaxation training alone[8] or there were no differences in efficacy between CBT and exposure therapy alone, in combination, or in combination with relaxation training.[6] The main components of CBT for GAD include:

- Psychoeducation
- Self-monitoring
- Relaxation training
- Cognitive restructuring
- Exposure to internal and external triggers of worry

The main goal of CBT is to alter the worry cycle present in GAD and to target the physical arousal, cognitions, and behavioral responses to worry. It is important to note, however, that in general GAD is difficult to treat because of the generalized and complex nature of this type of anxiety.

Psychoeducation provides information about anxiety, including where it develops, the costs and benefits of worry, physiological reactions, and how the worry cycle evolved. It also includes presentation of the treatment model and a description of the various components.

Self-monitoring is a key element requiring the patient to examine worry from a new perspective (i.e., as an observer). Several self-monitoring forms exist which include measures of daily anxiety on a Likert scale and thought or worry records specific to anxiety-provoking thoughts.

Relaxation training is introduced early in treatment because the typical patient with GAD experiences significant tension. It is also helpful when exposure techniques are initiated.

Cognitive restructuring occurs throughout treatment and focuses on helping the patient assess their misappraisal of situations (e.g., overestimating the likelihood of something bad happening, catastrophizing that they will not be able to cope).

Exposure involves working with the client to evoke images of their worries, hold them in mind for 30 minutes, and then generate as many alternative outcomes as possible.

Mr. X was introduced to the CBT model for GAD. Through psychoeducation, we discovered a long pattern of worrying that has likely affected his enjoyment of life and contributed to the high level of physical tension. We began monitoring his anxiety and identifying worry themes. Progressive muscle relaxation (PMR) was introduced in session and he was provided a compact disc recording of PMR to incorporate into his daily routine as a tool to cope with tension. We also examined his worries more closely and focused on breaking the cycle by exploring one specific worry for most of the session. This was followed by generating a list of alternative outcomes to his fear and worry. In addition, we helped Mr. X organize the multiple house repair projects and problem solve his difficulties at work. Owing to the significant stress in his life and concerns about his job performance, we discussed the possibility of adding medication to further improve his symptoms.

Combined Psychotherapy and Pharmacotherapy for Generalized Anxiety Disorder

There are conflicting reports about the efficacy of combined treatment for GAD. A meta-analysis performed on the small number of studies comparing combined treatments was inconclusive.[9] Other studies, however, reported that the combination of a BZD plus CBT produced a more rapid response.[10,11]

Introducing Combined Treatment

 Mr. X was presented with the latest information on the treatment of GAD. Following a discussion of treatment options and a risk–benefit analysis, he decided to begin CBT while we continued to explore the risks and benefits of medication.

Possible discussion points include:
- *Let us discuss the risks and benefits of medication.*
- *I think that medication may help with some of your anxiety but in the long-term, CBT can help you cope more effectively.*
- *Let us talk about the risks and benefits of combining treatments.*

Coordination of care is necessary for a successful treatment outcome. If more than one clinician is providing care, it is important for them to remain in contact during treatment. Following a signed release of information, there are several questions that may be useful, including:

Questions to ask the psychotherapist
- *What symptoms are you targeting?*
- *What specific worries have you been targeting?*
- *When do you plan to begin exposure?*
- *What is the best way to coordinate the medications with your work?*

Questions to ask the pharmacotherapist
- *What medications are you recommending?*
- *What symptoms are you targeting?*
- *What is your recommendation for the class of medication (e.g., BZD, AED, antidepressant [AD])?*

CLINICAL RECOMMENDATIONS

With mild levels of anxiety, we would initiate CBT if available and the patient is agreeable. With more severe, short-term anxiety, we would consider adding a BZD or pregabalin in addition to CBT. With more chronic anxiety, we would consider combining an AD or buspirone with psychotherapy, perhaps adding a BZD for short-term symptom relief while giving the primary course of medication and psychotherapy time to take full effect.

There are numerous self-help manuals available for patients and clinicians. Although there is little empirical support for these manuals, they may be useful and are very informative. These guides include *Mastery of Your Anxiety and Worry* by Zinbarg et al.[12]; *Natural Relief for Anxiety: Complimentary Strategies for Easing Fear, Panic and Worry* by Bourne et al.[13]; and *10 Simple Solutions to Worry* by Gyoerkoe and Wiegartz.[14]

Mr. X experienced a significant increase in symptoms when he was anxiety monitoring. Soon after CBT was initiated, he cancelled several appointments and felt overwhelmed with our focus on his worry. Eventually, he determined the benefits of medication outweighed the risks and he began a BZD (lorazepam 1 mg/b.i.d.). The medication was taken during times when his anxiety was high. It was also used during exposure. With the combination approach, Mr. X was able to utilize cognitive restructuring effectively as we continued to work through each of his worries. Although PMR was initially very difficult, he developed proficiency and incorporated it into his daily routine. We successfully problem solved ways to complete some of the house projects and set aside others without any additional worry. In addition, his performance at work improved although he continued to work long hours. Slowly his BZD use decreased as his coping skills increased and he continued CBT.

Figure 10-1 outlines the approach we would recommend for treatment of GAD.

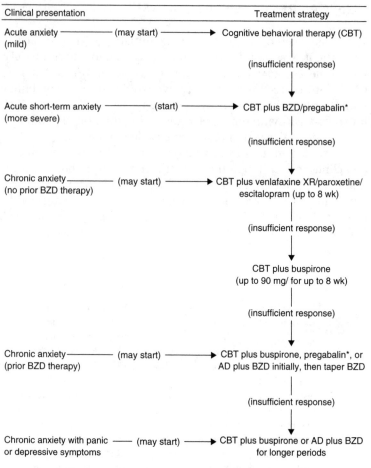

FIGURE 10-1 ▨ Treatment strategy for generalized anxiety disorder. CBT, cognitive behavioral therapy; BZD, benzodiazepine; XR, extended release; FDA, U.S. Food and Drug Administration. (Adapted from Janicak. *Principles and Practice of Psychopharmacotherapy*, 4th ed. Lippincott Williams and Wilkins, Philadelphia, PA, 2006.)

Learning points

- GAD is difficult to treat, but CBT has been shown to be effective.
- Various classes of psychotropics have demonstrated benefit for GAD.
- The benefit of combining pharmacotherapy and psychotherapy in GAD is less well studied but this approach may provide a faster resolution of symptoms.

REFERENCES

1. Mitte K. Meta-analysis of cognitive-behavioral treatments for generalized anxiety disorder: A comparison with pharmacotherapy. *Psychol Bull.* 2005;131(5):785–795.
2. Pollack MH, Zaninelli R, Goddard A, et al. Paroxetine in the treatment of generalized anxiety disorder: Results of a placebo-controlled, flexible-dosage trial. *J Clin Psychiatry.* 2001;62(5):350–357.
3. Stocchi F, Nordera G, Jokinen RH, et al. Paroxetine Generalized Anxiety Disorder Study team. Efficacy and tolerability of paroxetine for the long-term treatment of generalized anxiety disorder. *J Clin Psychiatry.* 2003;64(3):250–258.
4. Davidson JR. Pharmacotherapy of generalized anxiety disorder. *J Clin Psychiatry.* 2001;62(Suppl 11):46–50.
5. Gelenberg AJ, Lydiard RB, Rudolph RL, et al. Efficacy of venlafaxine extended-release capsules in nondepressed outpatients with generalized anxiety disorder: A 6-month randomized controlled trial. *JAMA.* 2000;283(23):3082.
6. Norton PJ, Price EC. A meta-analytic review of adult cognitive-behavioral treatment outcome across the anxiety disorders. *J Nerv Ment Dis.* 2007;195(6):521–531.
7. Borkovec TD, Ruscio AM. Psychotherapy for generalized anxiety disorder. *J Clin Psychiatry.* 2001;62(Suppl 11):37–42.
8. Siev J, Chambless DL. Specificity of treatment effects: Cognitive therapy and relaxation for generalized anxiety and panic disorders. *J Consult Clin Psychol.* 2007;75(4):513–522.
9. Bandelow B, Seidler-Brandler U, Becker A, et al. Meta-analysis of randomized controlled comparisons of psychopharmacological and psychological treatments for anxiety disorders. *World J Biol Psychiatry.* 2007;8(3):175–187.
10. Power KG, Simpson RJ, Swanson V, et al. A controlled comparison of cognitive-behaviour therapy, diazepam, and placebo alone or

in combination, for the treatment of generalised anxiety disorder. *J Anxiety Disord.* 1990a;4(4):267–292.

11. Power KG, Simpson RJ, Swanson V, et al. Controlled comparison of pharmacological and psychological treatment of generalized anxiety disorder in primary care. *Br J Gen Pract.* 1990b;40(336):289–294.

12. Zinbarg RE, Craske MG, Barlow DH. *Mastery of your anxiety and worry (MAW): therapist guide (treatments that work),* 2nd ed. New York: Oxford University Press; 2006.

13. Bourne EJ, Brownstein A, Garano L. *Natural relief for anxiety: complimentary strategies for easing fear, panic and worry.* Oakland: New Harbinger Publications; 2004.

14. Gyoerkoe KL, Wiegartz PS. *10 simple solutions to worry: how to calm your mind, relax your body and reclaim your life.* Oakland: New Harbinger Publications; 2006.

SUGGESTED READINGS

Barlow DH, ed. *Clinical handbook of psychological disorders,* 3th ed. New York: The Guilford Press; 2007:154–208.

Fisher JR, O'Donohue WT, eds. *Practitioner's guide to evidence-based psychotherapy.* New York, NY: Springer; 2006.

Janicak PG, Davis JM, Preskorn SH, et al. *Principles and practice of psychopharmacotherapy,* 4th ed. Philadelphia: Lippincott Williams & Wilkins; 2006.

Conclusion

Integrating psychological and biological treatments in clinical practice is a challenging task for many reasons. First, it takes years to establish the efficacy of one method of treatment (i.e., medication, psychotherapy, or a device-based therapy). Taking the next step (i.e., considering the differential risk–benefit ratio for monotherapy versus combined therapy) requires much more complicated study designs, resources, and the willingness to conduct trials of sufficient scope to answer these questions adequately. Second, while insurance companies use existing research in their decision-making process, fiscal concerns often dictate support for the less expensive strategy, which usually translates to reimbursing one treatment or the other rather than their combination. Third, vastly different, and at times competing, clinical backgrounds encourage the separation rather than the integration of different approaches. Finally, patients often present to clinicians with their own biases for or against a particular therapy and may resist recommendations inconsistent with their personal choices.

We believe, however, that the existing evidence often supports an integrated approach and this strategy should be utilized more frequently in clinical practice. In this context, training programs need to provide a multidisciplinary perspective (e.g., courses of sufficient depth on medications in psychology programs, courses on how to properly conduct CBT in psychiatry residency programs) so that future clinicians can better negotiate the use of combined treatment for their patients. Further, practitioners will need the background to adequately communicate with providers from different treatment orientations.

We reviewed the evidence for the use of psychotherapy; pharmacotherapy, and device-based therapies alone or in integrated treatment strategies for major depression, obsessive compulsive disorder, panic disorder, posttraumatic stress disorder, sleep disorders, schizophrenia, bipolar disorder, borderline personality disorder, and generalized anxiety disorder. Our goal was to concisely present the existing evidence and provide guidance on how to most effectively apply it. The choice of disorders was dictated in part by the adequacy of data and in part by the breadth of experience with these approaches in clinical practice. Our hope is to build sufficient confidence in the selection and negotiation of the best strategy (e.g., monotherapy, sequenced therapy, combined therapy) for the patient.

We recognize that the selection of topics in this book was based on our interpretation of the present state of knowledge. Further, these choices were tempered by the risk–benefit ratio of the various treatments. Most importantly, research will continue to reveal even better strategies for these and other disorders (e.g., social phobia) in the future. Therefore, clinicians must stay current regarding advances in these various treatment approaches.

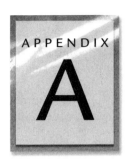

Websites

General

http://www.apa.org   American Psychological Association
http://www.psych.org   American Psychiatric Association
http://www.nimh.nih.gov   National Institute of Health
http://www.nmha.org   National Mental Health Organization
http://www.abct.org   Association for Behavioral and Cognitive
   Therapies
http://www.nami.org   National Alliance for the Mentally Ill
http://www.MayoClinic.com   Mayo Clinic
http://guidance.nice.org Britain's   National Institute for Clinical
   Excellence

Depression and Anxiety

http://www.depression.org   National Foundation for Depressive
   Illness
http://www.ocfoundation.org   Obsessive Compulsive
   Foundation
http://www.adaa.org   Anxiety Disorders Association of America
http://www.DBSAlliance.org   Depression and Support Alliance

Schizophrenia

http://www.narsad.org   National Alliance for Research on
   Schizophrenia and Depression

Borderline Personality Disorder

http://www.bpdcentral.com   Borderline Personality Disorder
Information and Support

http://www.borderlinepersonalitydisorder.com   National
Education Alliance for Borderline Personality Disorder

Glossary

AED	Antiepileptic drug
AD	Antidepressant
AE	Adverse effect
ASD	Acute distress disorder
ADHD	Attention deficit hyperactivity disorder
BDI-II	Beck Depression Inventory-II
BDNF	Brain-derived neurotrophic factor
BPD	Bipolar disorder
BT	Behavior therapy
BLT	Bright light therapy
BZD	Benzodiazepine
CATIE	Clinical Antipsychotic Treatment Intervention Effectiveness Study
CBT	Cognitive behavioral therapy
CBTp	Cognitive behavioral therapy for psychosis
CNS	Central nervous system
CPAP	Continuous positive airway pressure
CPT	Cognitive processing therapy
CRF	Corticotropin-releasing factor
CT	Cognitive therapy
DBS	Deep brain stimulation
DBT	Dialectical behavior therapy
DA	Dopamine
DSM-IV	Diagnostic and Statistical Manual, 4th edition
DVPX	Divalproex
EDS	Excessive daytime sleepiness
ECT	Electroconvulsive therapy
ERP	Exposure and response prevention
FDA	Food and Drug Administration
FFT	Family-focused therapy
FGA	First-generation antipsychotic
5-HT	Serotonin
GABA	Gamma-Aminobutyric acid

GAD	Generalized anxiety disorder
GLU	Glutamate
HPA	Hypothalamic-pituitary axis
IPT	Interpersonal therapy
IPSRT	Interpersonal social rhythm therapy
MAOI	Monoamine oxidase inhibitor
MBT	Mentalization-based therapy
MDQ	Mood Disorders Questionnaire
NE	Norepinephrine
NIMH	National Institute of Mental Health
NRI	Norepinephrine reuptake inhibitor
OSA	Obstructive sleep apnea
OCD	Obsessive compulsive disorder
OTC	Over-the-counter
PCP	Primary care physician
PD	Panic disorder
PMR	Progressive muscle relaxation
PRN	Take as needed
PTSD	Posttraumatic stress disorder
RLS	Restless legs syndrome
SAD	Seasonal affective disorder
SAMe	S-adenosyl methionine
SGA	Second-generation antipsychotic
SH	Sedative-hypnotics
SIT	Stress inoculation training
SRBD	Sleep-related breathing disorders
SNRI	Selective norepinephrine reuptake inhibitor
SRI	Serotonin reuptake inhibitor
SSRI	Selective serotonin reuptake inhibitor
STAR*D	Sequenced Treatment Alternatives for Resistant Depression Study
TCA	Tricyclic antidepressant
TMS	Transcranial magnetic stimulation
TRD	Treatment resistant depression
TSH	Thyroid-stimulating hormone
VNS	Vagus nerve stimulation
Y-BOCS	Yale-Brown Obsessive Compulsive Scale

Index